Younger Skin Starts
in the
GUT

Younger
Skin Starts
in the
GUT

4-Week Program to Identify and
Eliminate Your Skin-Aging Triggers—
Gluten, Wine, Dairy and Sugar

DR. NIGMA TALIB

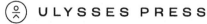 ULYSSES PRESS

Published in the US by:
ULYSSES PRESS
PO Box 3440
Berkeley, CA 94703
www.ulyssespress.com

ISBN: 978-1-61243-560-2
Library of Congress Control Number: 2015952143

First published in 2015 in the UK as *Reverse the Signs of Ageing* by Vermilion, an imprint of Ebury Publishing, part of the Penguin Random House group of companies

Printed in the United States

20 19 18 17 16 15 14 13 12 11 10 9 8 7

US acquisitions: Kelly Reed
US editor: Lauren Harrison
US proofreader: Renee Rutledge
Index: Sayre Van Young
Front cover design: Rebecca Lown
Front cover image: © Patrick Marks

CONTENTS

Foreword vii

Introduction.. 1

Are You Digest-Aging? 9

CHAPTER 1 Beauty Starts in the Gut... 13

CHAPTER 2 Eating Beauty... 48

CHAPTER 3 Inflammation—The Fire Within 82

CHAPTER 4 Rejuvenate Your Hormones..109

CHAPTER 5 The Beauty Prescription... 142

CHAPTER 6 Live an Age-Reversing Life...184

CHAPTER 7 The Age-Reversing Eating Plan 204

Afterword...262

Appendix: Putting It All into Practice—Your 12-Week Plan 263

Sources and References 267

Index 279

Dr. Nigma's Magic Nutritional Supplements 290

Acknowledgments..292

About the Author 295

FOREWORD

The gateway to our immune system is the skin. The largest organ in the human body is often ignored in the fight against disease. This "shield" is the first line of defense against inflammation and infection. Inflammation is the body's mechanism for self-protection. The goal is to remove toxic substances, including irritants, harmful pathogens and damaged cells. This is the first step in the healing process.

Improved health and a better quality of life can be achieved by addressing the underlying causes of inflammation and infection. Our bodies are aging faster than ever. Increased consumption of processed foods, sedentary lifestyles and overwhelming stress are feeding this process. This is leading to the epidemic growth of type 2 diabetes mellitus, obesity, heart disease and auto-immune conditions.

Now, Dr. Nigma Talib offers us an innovative solution to this problem through her groundbreaking book, *Younger Skin Starts in the Gut*. She utilizes her vast experience in treating thousands of patients over the past 14 years as a naturopathic doctor and medical aesthetician combined with the latest scientific research to formulate a better way to slow down the aging process.

Younger Skin Starts in the Gut is the easy-to-follow template for fixing your skin and combating the aging process. Dr. Talib builds this foundation to better health by working from the inside out. Remember, skin issues often serve as a warning sign to more significant medical conditions. First, Dr. Talib addresses "gut" health. She provides a view into the complexity of the digestive system and its trillions of bacteria. Current scientific research is focused on unearthing the "gut microbiome" and its relation to modern diseases. We already know the importance of these tiny bacteria and their critical role in the overall functioning of the human body. In fact, 70 percent of our immune system resides there.

The process begins through proper nutrition. A poor diet can lead to the spread of inflammation and infection. In the United States, the average adult consumes about 130 pounds of sugar every year. Increased consumption of sugar can lead to the production of advanced glycation end products. These harmful products can have a negative impact on aging and other chronic medical conditions. To protect your immune system, you must limit your consumption of sugar, gluten, cow's milk dairy and processed foods.

In *Younger Skin Starts in the Gut*, Dr. Talib helps sort through the confusion and misinformation of what to eat, and explains how it's important to choose foods that do something for you instead of something to you. Real foods provide the body with the nutrients needed to maintain proper skin health and function. Combine this with Dr. Talib's beauty prescription, and this program will help change your body on both a cellular and genetic level. This will not only reverse the signs of aging but also create a shield against future damage.

Younger Skin Starts in the Gut is a must read for any individual seeking a better solution to the aging process. How do I know this? I have witnessed the transformation of my patients who have used Dr. Talib's innovative inside-out approach to skin health.

Keith Berkowitz, M.D.
Medical Director, Center for Balanced Health
Author of *The Stubborn Fat Fix* and
The Complete Idiot's Guide to Flour-Free Eating

INTRODUCTION

How many times have you pooped today? Once, twice, not at all? Whatever your answer, I bet it wasn't the first question you were expecting to be asked when opening a book about reversing aging. But this is no ordinary beauty book. I don't believe that tackling aging or getting perfect skin is related solely to what you put on the outside of your body. It is also about what you put inside your body, as deep down inside the gut is where real aging begins.

I'm Dr. Nigma Talib, naturopathic doctor and medical aesthetician, and I've been helping patients with their health and beauty issues for 20 years in my clinics across the globe. During that time I've treated thousands of patients that all have one thing in common: they now look and feel younger (and healthier) than they would have done if they'd never come to see me. And by the end of this book, I'm hoping that's what's going to happen to you too.

ANTI-AGING FROM THE INSIDE

My story begins when I started my first practice in Vancouver back in 2001. I am a licensed naturopathic doctor (ND). This means I am qualified to treat the root cause of illness using a variety of safe and effective therapies, including acupuncture and Traditional Chinese Medicine, botanical medicine, clinical nutrition, homeopathy, lifestyle counseling and physical medicine. Naturopathic doctors treat a wide variety of chronic health conditions, such as allergies, chronic pain, digestive issues, hormonal imbalances, obesity, chronic fatigue and menopause—to name a few.

Naturopathic doctors are not the same as naturopaths. A licensed naturopathic doctor must have an undergraduate degree in pre-medical studies. We receive over 1,200 hours of clinical training and must treat over 225 patients before we even get our qualification. At a correctly accredited school, the naturopathic medicine curriculum receives significantly more hours in training in nutrition than graduates of some of the best medical schools in the US, if not the world, and a similar training in the biomedical sciences, which covers subjects such as anatomy, cell biology, physiology, neuroscience and biochemistry.[1]

This medical background meant that as soon as I opened the doors to my clinic, I started seeing patients with all sorts of health concerns. But as they'd talk about their symptoms, they wouldn't just talk about their health, but also about their appearance—and time after time they'd start telling me that they were aging faster than they thought they should. They were complaining of a lack of brightness in their face, skin texture getting rougher, fine lines and wrinkles appearing faster than they expected or developing a noticeable increase in pigmentation. Some had gotten to the point where they felt, "Well, I am getting older, so I guess I should accept that I feel and look worse than I did when I was in my 20s." Others were using fillers and face-freezing jabs to try to disguise the problems they were seeing, believing that this was their only option to try to change what was happening. I disagreed. Yes, there is a pressure on women and men to look younger, but it didn't make sense to me to be exhausted on the inside and older on the outside, masking both with fillers and paralyzing injections.

Seems I was right. As their medical treatment progressed and we addressed the gut problems, hormonal imbalances or inflammation behind pretty much all of their health concerns, my patients also started to notice major skin changes; it was improving in all the aging areas they had been complaining about before. They were thrilled—and so was I. Not only was I helping my patients achieve optimum wellness, I was also helping them turn back the clock and look better than they ever had before. Soon they started to tell their friends and family what I was doing, and once their husbands noticed the change I had them coming in as well! No wonder I think of my patients as one big happy family.

At this point, to complement my ND qualification I decided to also train as a medical aesthetician: a skincare specialist who can use medical-like treatments. I felt that together, the two could help me absolutely determine the root causes of why people age before they should.

I saw more and more patients, and as my knowledge grew, I could clearly see the link between their health and why they were aging. Eventually it got to a point where I realized there was a clear correlation between a change in the health of someone's gut or their diet and their skin. For example, if someone had been eating more dairy in the weeks before they saw me they'd often appear with dark circles under their eyes; a higher intake of alcohol would leave skin with more fine lines and wrinkles around their mouth, the nasolabial folds (the lines that come down the sides of your nostrils to your mouth) and the eye area; if I took gluten out of a patient's diet, in no time it would result in a face that was less bloated and puffy.

I used this in combination with traditional Chinese face-mapping to create treatment plans. I quickly realized that following my plan helped my patients' skin clear up and reversed many of those signs of aging they were worried about. Patients with rosacea, redness, pigmentation problems and dull, dry or sagging skin noticed such considerable changes that their friends and family were asking if they'd had some work done! It was so powerful that I couldn't understand why all dermatologists weren't using dietary changes to treat the root cause of distressed skin or as an anti-aging weapon.

The final piece of the puzzle

I consider myself a biochemical detective, always trying to find the true root cause of my patients' problems rather than just treating their symptoms with a plaster-like approach. I realized at this point that all of the evidence was pointing to one thing behind the premature aging—and many of the other health and skin issues my clients were complaining of—and that was poor digestive function.

This might surprise you; after all, how can something that goes on deep inside the body, far, far away from your face reflect how old you look or how healthy your skin appears? But it didn't surprise me. The gut is the control center of the body, the place where health and death begins. Whatever happens in the gut will show up in the skin and dictate the health of your entire body. I'll explain more thoroughly how this can be over the pages that follow, but, very briefly, this is what happens: poor health within the gut starves the skin of the nutrients it needs to thrive; it causes an increase of inflammatory molecules in the body that directly and indirectly attack the skin, which causes faster aging and aggravates inflammatory skin conditions, such as acne and rosacea. An imbalanced or unhealthy gut can also affect many of the hormones in the body, which again has an effect on the skin. In a nutshell, poor gut health is behind at least three of the fundamental mechanisms controlling how fast or slow your skin, and your body, will age. I realized that by treating the health of the gut and restoring good digestive function, as I was doing now in all my patients, I was tackling these aging triggers and creating the amazing effects we both could see.

I didn't really have a name for what I was seeing until one day I was treating a patient who had digestive problems. She was also concerned about her skin and how she was looking older, and I said, "Well, you do know that your digestion problems mean you're aging faster?" She replied, "You mean I'm digest-aging." All of a sudden I had a name for what I was seeing in so many people. The circle was complete—I knew what was causing it, I knew how to tackle it and now I had a name to explain it to the world.

Since then, I have treated literally thousands of patients for digest-aging and I am confident that the beauty and health worlds have missed something. I mention health here because of course the skin isn't the only thing that shows signs of aging, and the gut can also be the root cause of many of the other issues that plague the body as we get older. Aching joints, weight gain around the middle, thinning hair, poor sleep, lack of energy and the severity of menopausal symptoms can also all be related to gut health. Get your gut healthy and these symptoms can also improve. No wonder that after treatment my patients not only *look* younger, but say they *feel* younger too, as everything seems to improve about their health—they regain their energy and get a spring in their step.

ANTI-AGING FROM THE OUTSIDE

So does this mean you should throw away your skin creams and never have another face treatment in your life? No! The best skin comes from treating the inside *and* the outside. The outside needs topical treatments to strengthen and hydrate the skin, stimulate collagen, fade pigmentation or reduce fine lines and wrinkles, but combining this with healing the body from within creates the perfect marriage of techniques. But with so many lotions, potions, treatments and injections available to us today, all claiming to work miracles, how do you know which are going to give you the best result? Well, later on in this book I'll explain that too, sharing exactly what I use directly on my patients—many of whom are A-list actresses, actors and models whose faces are their fortune.

What I do believe, though, is that the obviously worked-on face, where someone has overdone the fillers so everything is just a little bit puffy, or where they've had so much face-freezing they can no longer make the natural expressions that are our first signs of communication, is the "new old." I'm not alone—more and more of my patients are increasingly rejecting injectables and instead are turning to anti-aging treatments that deliver more natural results—those that result in fresh, radiant skin at the cellular level and still allow the face to have expression.

The way I see it, the "new youth" is to have clear, glowing, bright, dewy, even-toned, firm skin. You want to make healthier what you already have so that when people look at your skin they don't think you are "xx" years old, but instead think, "Wow, that person looks glowing." Yes, you might have a few lines showing a life well lived, but you don't have to have rough skin or excessive sagging to go with them—and you can have amazing skin texture, a brightness to your skin and minimal pigmentation whatever your age. What I'm saying is that while some aging is natural and unavoidable, as far as I'm concerned if you take control of your health, premature aging is optional.

This is what I've been saying to my patients for years now and I'm thrilled that writing this book allows me to be able to share this knowledge with a much wider audience than I could ever see personally in my clinics. Think of this book as kind of like having me as your personal naturopathic doctor in your home wherever you are in the world.

HOW THE BOOK WORKS

The advice I give over the pages that follow will help you pinpoint the root causes of premature aging—and then show you how to reverse them. There are plans to tackle four main areas that I now believe absolutely to be behind the symptoms of poor health and premature aging. The plans work in three stages—Clear, Correct and Protect (CCP), with options to "Power Up" throughout if you want an added boost.

- In Chapter 1, the Gut-Balancing CCP Plan tackles the health of the gut.
- In Chapter 3, the Inflammation-Fighting CCP Plan tackles the epidemic of inflammation affecting our cells.

• In Chapter 4, the Hormone-Balancing CCP Plan tackles the hormone imbalances that are leaving us looking and feeling frazzled.

• In Chapter 5, the Skincare CCP Plan tackles skincare, ensuring it is just as effective as we hope.

As you'll discover, all of these are closely interlinked and for that reason I strongly urge you to read the book as a whole before you start making any changes—and that you follow the plans in turn, rather than attempting to pick and choose the advice you use. At the end of the book, you'll find a guide to how to put it all into practice stage by stage, week by week.

So what do the plans aim to do? Simply, they fight those primary aging triggers using a mix of dietary changes, lifestyle changes, evidence-based skincare and some highly targeted supplementation. We start with the health of the gut, as it's my absolute belief that this is where aging begins. I'm then going to reveal how what you eat might impact how fast you age—and, more surprisingly, how some simple changes could eliminate lines, wrinkles and under-eye bags in a matter of weeks.

I'll talk about inflammation, the silent epidemic aging so many of our bodies today, and then move on to why all of the above combined with modern life might be throwing your hormones into chaos.

Add to this my little black book of skincare secrets, advice on lifestyle changes that turn back time and the Age-Reversing Eating Plan packed with delicious recipes, which I guarantee will trigger changes in your skin if you follow it, and the pages that follow really are a complete anti-aging makeover unlike any other you've tried before! In summary:

The eight signs of aging this plan can fight:

1   Fine lines and wrinkles

2   Sagging skin

3   Uneven skin tone

4   Dull, lifeless skin

5   Rough skin texture

6   Adult acne

7   Rosacea

8   Under-eye circles and bags

The four ways it does it:

1   Improves the health of your gut, the place where aging begins

2   Fights inflammation to combat aging at a deep, cellular level

3   Balances the youth-boosting and aging hormones that modern life disrupts

4   Reveals the ultimate anti-aging skincare regime

The one amazing result:

A younger, healthier you

ARE YOU DIGEST-AGING?

Before I move on to *how*, let me give you a clear reason *why* you should make these changes and reveal just how much you might be digest-aging.

The symptoms below are all possible signs that your digestion isn't working as well as it could. Check as many that apply, and then see what that says about you.

Checklist 1: Digestive issues

Check the box if you find yourself suffering from the symptom:

- ❏ Acid reflux
- ❏ Bloating after meals
- ❏ Burping
- ❏ Constipation
- ❏ Diarrhea
- ❏ Flatulence
- ❏ Heartburn/indigestion
- ❏ Incomplete evacuation (small, pebble-like stools)
- ❏ Less than one bowel movement a day
- ❏ Rectal itching
- ❏ Undigested food in your stool

Checklist 2: Skin problems

Check the box if you've noticed the skin signs worsening faster than you might expect, considering your age and skin protection habits— or if you think you are experiencing any of the below to a greater extent than peers of the same age:

- ❑ Acne
- ❑ Blackheads
- ❑ Bumpy skin
- ❑ Dry skin
- ❑ Dullness
- ❑ Eczema
- ❑ Fine lines and wrinkles
- ❑ Loose, sagging skin, on, for example, the jowls
- ❑ Open, enlarged pores
- ❑ Pigmentation
- ❑ Reddening of the skin
- ❑ Rosacea
- ❑ Rough skin texture

Checklist 3: Health concerns

Check the box if you regularly suffer any of the following:

- ❑ Cracking nails or vertical ridges on the nails
- ❑ Fatigue
- ❑ Feeling cold
- ❑ Foggy brain
- ❑ Food intolerances
- ❑ Frequent minor infections, such as coughs and colds
- ❑ Fungal infections
- ❑ Joint pains
- ❑ Menstrual cramps

❑ Menstrual irregularities
❑ PMS
❑ Sleep problems
❑ Slow weight loss
❑ Sugar cravings
❑ Thinning hair or hair loss
❑ Thrush
❑ Weight gain
❑ White coating on the tongue

What do your results reveal?

The more symptoms that you checked, the greater the chance that you are digest-aging—but what's also important is exactly *which* of the sections you checked.

If you have a clear majority of symptoms in checklist 1, you have a low level of digest-aging. That's good, kind of ... While it does show that your digestion is upset in some way, it means it's not yet noticeably starting to impact on the rest of your body. If you tackle whatever is causing the digest-aging now, you'll probably find it never will—plus you'll be free of those uncomfortable, annoying digestive issues you pinpointed.

If you marked symptoms mostly in checklists 1 and 2, you have a moderate level of digest-aging. This means there's a good chance that the concerns you have regarding your skin are linked to issues causing your gut symptoms too. Using solutions that heal and calm the gut and tackling skin issues with the right topical treatments will probably turn things around completely for you.

If you marked symptoms in all three checklists, you have a high level of digest-aging. Again, your gut alone could be behind everything you are suffering, but it's going to be particularly important for you to also follow the specific anti-inflammatory and hormone-balancing plans.

If you marked symptoms mostly in checklists 2 and 3, you have a low to moderate level of digest-aging. While you might be unhappy with your skin, it's possible that your digestion alone might not be behind the problems you have. They may be more related to inflammation or hormonal imbalances, or to not using the right skincare. However, I'd still suggest you follow the Gut-Balancing CCP Plan that you will find in Chapter 1 on page 37. Because we are so used to our bodies and their quirks, many of us don't realize our gut is imbalanced until we improve its health and suddenly discover how a healthy gut should behave.

If you mostly marked checklists 1 and 3, you have a moderate level of digest-aging. You are, however, lucky that it hasn't yet shown up that much on your skin. This could be because you have extremely good genetics, or perhaps your suncare or skincare regimen is mitigating some of the damage you'd normally be seeing. The fact that you are suffering from gut symptoms, though, does mean your gut is out of balance, and by improving that and working on lowering inflammation and rebalancing your hormone levels, you'll keep your skin looking good.

If you didn't mark anything, then why are you reading this book?! Go and do something else. Actually don't—modern life, as you'll see, is putting your whole body under pressure every single day and while you might have escaped so far, you can still learn how to protect yourself in the future.

So, now, let's get started by looking at *exactly* why the gut is the foundation of healthy aging and how, if it's not healthy, it can wreak havoc with so much of your body, making you old before your time.

CHAPTER 1

BEAUTY STARTS IN THE GUT

It's not an exaggeration to say that I look to the gut when it comes to treating every patient I see; it really is the control center for the entire body. Anything that goes wrong in the gut will cause symptoms all over your body—and it will absolutely show as problems on your face, sooner or later. To beat premature aging, you have to take care of your gut. Or, as I say to my patients, a problem in your bowels will eventually create jowls.

This might surprise you—after all, most of us think that the job of the gut is merely to digest our food and eliminate waste, but it's far more complex than that. The digestive system covers a huge area within the body—in 2014, using the most sophisticated techniques so far, experts at Sweden's Sahlgrenska Academy in Gothenburg measured it to be about 16½ ft (5 m) long and its surface area, if you managed to separate it all out, would cover an area around 323–430 sq ft (30–40 sq m), the size of a small studio apartment.[1] Yes, that is all squished up inside your body. Inside, predominantly in the large intestine, live around 100 trillion bacteria. They're so plentiful they outnumber our body's cells here 10 to 1—meaning, if you think about it, we're only 10 percent human and 90 percent bacteria. If you managed to scoop out all that bacteria and place them in a jar, it would weigh around 3 lb (1.4 kg).

These tiny bacteria are now emerging as one of the major control systems of our entire body. They may be small but they are very powerful. If they are in balance, you are more likely to be in better health—you'll find it easier to control your weight, and you'll have healthier, more youthful-looking skin. Why? Because those bacteria have a direct role to play in the health of that skin. For example, they create and help you assimilate nutrients the skin needs to protect itself and repair; they protect the integrity of the gut lining, which helps fight inflammation that ages skin; and they play a role in protecting the skin against damage—both from toxins created within our own body and those created by external factors, such as UV light and pollution. The gut bacteria can also affect acne as the gut, brain and skin produce a neuropeptide called Substance P, which affects sebum production. In one Russian study looking at a group of patients with acne, 54 percent of them had what the researchers referred to as "impaired" gut bacteria.[2] So many skin conditions can be linked right back to this one source.

FEELINGS—SO MUCH MORE THAN FEELINGS

There's also an important connection between the gut and the emotions—it's no coincidence that people say "I have a gut feeling about this," or they suffer loose bowels if they are nervous about something. The brain and the gut communicate thousands of times every single day. Your gut, in fact, is your second brain. It contains an estimated 500 million neurons and releases at least 40 different neurotransmitters; 95 percent of the body's serotonin (a hormone associated with improved mood but that also controls gut contraction) is found within the gut, and you have more serotonin receptors in your gut than your brain. We also know that while the brain sends signals to the gut, for every one message it sends down, the gut sends nine messages back, covering everything from how full you feel to whether it's time to go to the bathroom. And, just recently, it's also been discovered the gut can affect emotions. It's now believed that certain pathogens in the gut produce substances that can trigger symptoms of anxiety and possibly even depression-like symptoms in people who carry them. I always love it when research and clinical practice show the same thing, as for years now I have seen evidence of this. I have often found that my patients who have anxiety and depression-like symptoms also have digestive issues, and once we get to the root cause of those, the anxiety and low mood also lift. Conversely, though, favorable bacteria can help create more positive emotions: French research published in the *British Journal of Nutrition*,[3] for example, found that women supplementing with a product called Probio-Stick containing two specific strains of bacteria (*Lactobacillus Rosell-52* and *Bifidobacterium Rosell-175*) felt less anxious during periods of stress. Why do we care about any of this? Because emotions are also strongly linked to skin health and the speed at which we age. One study on identical twins, for example, found that the twin who had experienced more stress in her life (the doctors chose twins where one was divorced and one was happy in her relationship) looked on average 2 years older than her less-pressured sister.[4] I've seen patients that look 4, 5, even 10 years older than their chronological age because of the stress that they have gone through in their life.

THE DIGEST-AGING CONNECTION

The idea that the gut and aging were linked was first suggested back in the 19th century when the Russian biologist Dr. Ilya Mechnikov realized that the Bulgarian population, a particularly long-living and healthy people at the time, consumed high quantities of yogurt. He had long suspected that toxins emitted by some of the more negative bacteria in the gut might aggravate the aging process, but he then started to suspect that the bacteria in the fermented milk so beloved in the Bulgarian diet might counteract this. He took his research into the laboratory and realized that, yes, the bacteria in the yogurt did seem to prevent the more harmful bacteria in the gut from releasing their toxins.

Mechnikov's work was the foundation of the science of probiotics—something I regularly add to the daily diet of my patients to help tackle digest-aging. But there's a lot more to tackling the gut-aging connection than just adding probiotics. Over the years, studying thousands of patients, I've identified four main reasons why the skin might age prematurely if the gut is imbalanced, and you need to counteract them all. Before I go into them in detail, though, there's something I need to point out.

In this chapter, I'm about to cover each gut problem separately. If only it were that simple. In reality, all the problems are usually linked to each other and also to the other core aging triggers—inflammation and hormonal imbalance. If you have one of these problems, you either already have at least one of the others, or they are waiting around the corner if you don't do something to stop them. To make it simpler, think of your gut as performing like a symphony orchestra: when everything is in time, it makes beautiful synchronized music; if, however, one member of that orchestra goes out of sync, they'll play out of time on their own for a little while, but eventually they will start to impact some of the other musicians, who will start to skip beats too. Eventually you're making a horrible noise rather than beautiful music—until the conductor gets control of things again. That's also what happens with the gut; for example, if you're not digesting food correctly, the by-products that form as food ferments in the gut damages the gut bacteria and affects the gut lining (causing a problem called leaky gut—see page 26). If leaky gut occurs, you absorb fewer nutrients and it becomes easier for bad bacteria to adhere to the bowel wall. At this point, the good bacteria start to be crowded out, and this causes even less nutrient absorption and further problems with fermentation. The problems just keep escalating, unless you, the conductor, take control again.

PROBLEM 1: MALABSORPTION AND MALDIGESTION

- **Why it causes aging:** Malabsorption and maldigestion reduce the supply of vitamins, minerals, proteins and antioxidants your skin needs to thrive.

- **Possible results:** Poor collagen renewal and hardening of the elastin fibers, leading to lines and wrinkles; increased inflammation in the skin, which is linked to rapid aging, acne and rosacea; roughness, dark circles and lowered circulation to the skin, which impact on brightness and skin tone.

Even if you eat the healthiest diet on the planet, how do you know if you are actually absorbing the nutrients you consume?

The simplest reason that the skin might be affected by gut problems is that they can interfere with the amount of nutrients you can absorb. Virtually every mineral and vitamin we eat aids the skin in some way—for example, vitamins C and E are imperative for collagen formation and repair, while the mineral zinc helps fight problems such as acne. If you're not absorbing those nutrients, guess what? They can't do their job and your skin will start to suffer. Protein absorption can also be affected by poor digestion—and protein is the building block of your skin, hair and nails. If you're not absorbing protein, you're going to see that reflected back when you look in the mirror. When nutrient absorption is impaired, you could be eating a diet packed with foods that are known to help create beautiful skin, such as berries, avocados and oily fish, but barely any of their vital vitamins, minerals or fatty acids are going to be absorbed.

Your gut bacteria also make nutrients. They make vitamin B7 (also known as biotin), a nutrient essential for cell renewal and healthy skin, hair and nails. They make vitamin B12, which carries oxygenated blood around the body, giving skin a youthful glow that money can't buy and face freezers, face fillers or even surgery can't achieve. Finally, bacteria help us make vitamin K, which helps prevent calcium attaching to the elastin fibers of the skin, keeping them springy and firm. If the gut bacteria aren't doing their job well, you'll be lacking in sufficient levels of all of those nutrients and your skin will prematurely suffer and sag.

This lack of nutrients also has the potential to reduce hormone levels in the body. I'll talk further about why good hormone balance is essential for healthy aging later in Chapter 4, but, for now, know that your body needs nutrients, such as the B vitamins and the minerals selenium and iodine, to help it manufacture hormones, such as estrogen, progesterone and thyroxine—all of which are vital for healthy, young-looking skin.

There are two main causes of poor nutrient absorption: malabsorption, where a problem in the digestive system stops the body from absorbing the nutrients from your food; and maldigestion, where you don't break down the food well enough to extract all you need from it. The two conditions often go hand in hand—and they are both something I see day in and day out in my practice.

How poor digestion ages you

The process of digestion starts as soon as you put something in your mouth. As you chew, saliva is released and this contains the enzyme ptyalin that starts to break down any carbohydrates you're consuming. When you swallow, the food passes down the esophagus and into the stomach. Here stomach acids and the enzyme pepsin should be waiting to start breaking down the protein that you've eaten. Within a few hours, food moves to the small intestine, where the majority of nutrients get absorbed via enzymes released from the pancreas. Finally, the food moves into the large intestine, where those all-important gut bacteria get to work making nutrients, but also further breaking down any leftover carbohydrates, fiber and even waste products such as dead cells to create vital by-products called short-chain fatty acids. Eventually, when that's all done and all that is left is waste the body can't use, the gut sends signals to the brain triggering you to visit the bathroom.

So what can go wrong during this process and why? A lot, is the answer. Let's take it step by step:

In the mouth: Many of us eat too quickly—we eat on the run, at our desk while fielding phone calls, or we snatch something seconds before we fly out of the door. As such, we tend to bolt our food down without adequately chewing it. This reduces how much saliva comes into contact with food and so carbohydrates, which normally begin to digest here in the mouth, can enter the system without going through the first step that starts their breakdown. This can make them harder to tackle effectively further down the line. And by carbohydrates I don't just mean foods such as rice, bread or pasta—fruits and vegetables are also carbohydrates. By not chewing well, you run the risk of a suboptimal digestion of essential skin nutrients, such as vitamin C, betacarotene (which converts into the vitamin A our skin needs) and the antioxidants that counteract the environmental damage from things such as pollutants and UV rays that make our skin age.

In the stomach: Not chewing food also slows things here. As food hits receptors in the cheeks and tongue, the brain starts to analyze exactly which of the macronutrients—protein, carbohydrates or fat—is in the mouthful that you're consuming. When it detects protein, it signals your stomach to start secreting the acid and pepsin you need to digest it. This is essential when it comes to skin health, as protein contains the amino acids that are the building blocks of our skin's foundations. If protein absorption is impaired, you'll notice your skin starts to lose its glow as cell turnover slows down. Lines and wrinkles form faster as daily damage is less likely to be repaired. Protein also builds hair and nails—a classic sign I notice in my patients when protein absorption is low is that their hair and nails don't seem to grow as fast.

Micronutrients, such as zinc, selenium and copper, are also essential for skin health and slowing down aging—copper, for example, works with zinc to help form collagen, and selenium is an antioxidant that helps fight against oxidation that causes skin damage—and absorption of these micronutrients can also be reduced if levels of acidity in your stomach are lowered.

But less surprising though—aging can also cause digest-aging! Production of both stomach acid and the enzymes we need for digestion declines as we age. It's funny, as we get older we often end up with problems with excess acid, which we treat with medication such as Pepto-Bismol, but your stomach needs to be acidic to digest food.

Hypochlorhydria—aka low stomach acid

If you have gas, bloating, burping after meals, a feeling that food just sits in the stomach, heartburn, bad breath, foul-smelling bowel movements and a regularly upset stomach, then it's possible your stomach acid levels are low. Another way to tell is to drink baking soda in water. It's not a foolproof test, but can give an indication that something is wrong. First thing in the morning before you have anything to eat or drink, add a quarter of a teaspoon of baking soda to a glass of water. Drink this down in one go—then see what happens. If you have healthy levels of stomach acid, you should burp within two to three minutes as the alkaline soda mixes with your stomach acid and creates carbon dioxide. If you don't burp, there's a good chance there's not enough acid there to cause a reaction.

Now if you're one of the many people reading this who regularly suffers from heartburn, indigestion or acid reflux, you might think there's no reason for you to carry out the test—after all, surely you've got too much acid? Don't be so sure. One cause of the conditions we think are "acidic" can actually be low stomach acid, which causes the stomach contents to remain within the stomach longer than they should. If you regularly suffer from these issues you should definitely check your acidity levels, but do note that if you are taking antacids or proton pump inhibitors to keep things under control, these will skew the results slightly. Ask your doctor if it's okay to stop the medication for a couple of days, and then try the test.

In the small intestine: When food moves to the small intestine, enzymes excreted by the pancreas take over the task of digestion— these are lipase, which acts on fat; amylase, which breaks down carbohydrates; and protease, which breaks down protein. As with stomach acid, enzyme production in the small intestine can also start to decline as we age. In fact, when French researchers checked enzyme levels in the population, they found that production increased until people reached their 30s—then it tapered back off again.[5] This lack of enzymes can quite clearly affect the skin in many ways—low levels of protease can cause poor protein digestion, with all those effects I mentioned before. Low amylase means fewer nutrients taken from carbohydrates, and if fat digestion is affected you don't break the fat down into the glycerols you need to absorb the fat-soluble vitamins A, D, E and K, and they'll just pass right out of your system in the stool. All of the fat-soluble nutrients are vital for skin health—vitamin A, for example, helps improve cell turnover, so if levels are low your skin will look and feel rough, even scaly; vitamin E is involved in the synthesis of collagen and helps protect skin against environmental damage; while low levels of vitamin D have been linked to the development of dark circles under the eyes. If you want good skin, you have to digest fat efficiently.

Admittedly your body does try to fight back against poor digestion—if food arrives in the small intestine partially digested, the pancreas tries to combat this by releasing higher levels of those vital enzymes. The problem is, just as you get a little burned out working too hard day in and day out, so does the pancreas, and eventually a problem called pancreatic insufficiency can develop. Many conventional doctors only treat this when it manifests in its most severe form, associated with problems like alcoholism or Crohn's disease, but as a naturopathic doctor I recognize what's called subclinical versions of many health problems. Conventional medicine doesn't address these concerns because they aren't life-threatening—but when an organ stops performing optimally it harms the health and prematurely ages the body. So why wait for it to worsen further before attempting to correct it?

Symptoms of low enzyme levels, which if left uncorrected may then develop into pancreatic insufficiency, include bloating or stomach pain after meals, production of excessive gas via belching or odorous flatulence, watery stools and signs of undigested food in your stools. If you regularly suffer these symptoms, you might want to ask a naturopathic doctor or other integrative medical professional for a test that checks your levels of substances called pancreatic elastase or chymotrypsin. These are both enzymes produced by the pancreas and if levels are low you will need to supplement to make up the deficit (see Power Up on page 41).

In the large intestine: Here it's the gut bacteria that do the majority of the work. I've already told you that these produce many of our B vitamins and vitamin K, therefore it's clear that if your bacteria is out of balance, the levels of the nutrients you produce might be lower than optimum. If the gut bacteria are out of balance, the lining of the gut can also be damaged, which in turn impacts on the levels of nutrients you can absorb. But on top of this, the bacteria also produce substances called short-chain fatty acids (SCFAs). These are vital for gut health. They provide the energy your gut runs on, and they help protect the colon lining and dramatically lower the risk of leaky gut syndrome (see page 26). They are extremely underrated contributors to your body's health.

But SCFAs are also essential for skin health and reversing aging. Specifically they help counteract inflammation. Inflammation is such a fundamental cause of aging and I have dedicated all of Chapter 3 to explaining why it's so important and how to fight it. For now, though, I will just say that if your body cannot fight inflammation you will be aging faster from within. You'll also be more prone to skin problems, such as acne, rosacea, eczema and psoriasis.

PROBLEM 2: DYSBIOSIS— AKA OUT-OF-BALANCE BACTERIA

- **Why it causes aging:** The bacteria in the gut normally produce vitamins that aid skin health and help with the absorption of nutrients from our food. Bacteria also create fatty acids that fight inflammation that ages our skin. If bacteria levels are low, not only does this conversion not happen but bacteria that release inflammatory substances are more likely to thrive. Bacteria also play a role in protecting the skin against damage from UV rays and other harmful factors.

- **Possible results:** Dry, papery skin due to lower levels of the lipids that aid hydration; puffiness around the eyes and jowls caused by fluid linked to inflammation; lines, wrinkles and pigmentation caused by more rapid damage from UV rays, pollutants and oxidants.

If you want younger-looking skin, you must look after the bacteria that populate the gut. They are fundamental in determining how fast, and how well, you age.

As I said before, the gut contains around 100 trillion bacteria, a collection also known as the microbiome or microbiota. Which types you have of the 100,000 different strains discovered so far is as individual as your fingerprint, but as a general rule, a healthy microbiome should contain at least 400 different strains of bacteria, and 85 percent of those should be ones that help the body function positively in some way. Studies, however, are showing that this isn't always the case. A 2013 study from the University of Copenhagen,[6] for example, found that almost a quarter of people they studied had 40 percent fewer bacteria than would normally be expected in a healthy gut—and the bugs they did have were more likely to be prone to causing inflammation than the health-promoting bacteria that fight it.

There are many reasons why our microbiome is suffering and they begin as early as birth. Babies in the womb only have a very limited microbiome, but get a huge "injection" of bacteria as they travel through the vaginal canal during birth; however, babies delivered by Cesarean section don't get that exact same boost. Breastfed babies also have a more diverse microbiome than those fed on formula. These early years are so important that scientists now believe that while we can tweak the microbiome in adulthood, its fundamental makeup could be set as early as the age of three.

We also live in a more sterile world now and this reduces the amount of diversity within our gut. Our clean houses and better food hygiene mean we just don't expose our bodies to as many types of bacteria as before (in years gone by our food would naturally contain dirt and molds that exposed us to a greater diversity of bacteria). Then there are our lifestyles—stress, alcohol, commonly used medications, such as non-steroidal anti-inflammatory drugs, and our diets can determine whether our bacteria is mostly formed of healthy bacteria, or the opposite. A recent trial at Harvard University,[7] for example, found that adapting the diet to one focused on fruits, vegetables and whole grains can increase levels of bacteria that dampen inflammation in as little as 24 hours. Conversely, a trial at Ohio State University[8] showed that during stress, more inflammation-producing bacteria started to thrive—and good bacteria started to disappear.

Then there are antibiotics. There's no doubt that antibiotics save lives, but taking them is like setting off a bomb to destroy a tin can. Yes, they'll kill the bacteria that are making you sick, but they'll also wipe out bacteria indiscriminately around the body, including the health-promoting bacteria that live in the gut. Most of these repopulate within a week of your finishing the course of antibiotics, but recent research has shown that in some people the microbiome changes slightly forever.[9]

When any of these things start to interfere with the health of the good bacteria, bad bacteria can start to thrive. The reason why is simple: imagine your gut as a street—when they are performing well, good bacteria produce levels of lactic acid and fatty acids that make the neighborhood an unappealing place for the bad bacteria to live. If the numbers of good bacteria start to decline, however, those acid levels also decline and the bad bacteria start to move in—next thing you know, they've multiplied and are starting to take over. That's dysbiosis: when the number of the bad bacteria starts to outbalance the good. It's a state that up to one in four of us, if the Copenhagen trial translates to the population at large (and the researchers felt it would), are currently living in.

How dysbiosis ages you

Remember, without the right types of bacteria you can't make the nutrients the skin needs and you'll be more likely to have bacteria that trigger inflammation that directly ages the skin. If you have an overgrowth of bad bacteria, the waste products they excrete—their poop, if you like—also create all kinds of internal toxins that add to this inflammatory cascade. Because your levels of bacteria that produce the fatty acids that help naturally combat that inflammation are being crowded out, your ability to fight back declines.

The gut bacteria are also involved in how hormones are processed in the body, and, as any woman who has broken out in blemishes the week before her period knows, hormones can create chaos in the skin. Like inflammation, hormonal imbalances and the production of what I refer to as "dirty hormones" in the body is another issue that must be addressed if you want to age well (which I'm going to cover extensively in Chapter 4), but balancing hormones begins in the gut and it begins by ensuring a healthy balance of gut bacteria.

So what happens if you alter the gut bacteria and create a more favorable microbiome? In my patients I find skin becomes smoother and more hydrated, fine lines and wrinkles can start to disappear and the overall skin tone improves. But you don't just have to take my word for it. Altering the microbiome is not just an area that I am interested in; it's also one cosmetic companies are intrigued by. This means not only do I have the experience of my patients to show me there are clear benefits to their skin when you favorably tweak bacteria levels, there are published studies that can help me confirm it too. Here are just three that show what happens:

One study[10] found that giving people a supplement of a strain of *Lactobacillus* helps improve the skin's immune response to UV light—one of the most important contributors to premature aging. This shows that if you have the right gut bacteria in your system, your skin can better defend itself against sun damage.

In another study[11] the researchers tested whether a strain of probiotic in the *Lactobacillus* family helped improve the barrier function of the skin. It did. Not only did this decrease skin sensitivity, but it could help reduce damage to the skin by pollutants and toxins that cause more rapid aging.

A further trial[12] showed that 24 weeks of consuming a drink containing three different types of probiotic—along with some other healthy skin boosters—helped reduce water loss from the skin and boosted the skin barrier in women who had sensitive, dry skin.

These studies show clearly that taking steps to help rebalance the types and numbers of gut bacteria, so the gut becomes a place where good bacteria thrive and the more harmful bacteria don't feel at home, is a vital step to fight premature aging.

PROBLEM 3: LEAKY GUT

- **Why it causes aging:** Leaky gut triggers the release of inflammatory substances into the bloodstream that damage the skin. It overloads the entire body systematically, affects the liver by preventing it from processing hormones correctly and lowers the levels of nutrients absorbed via the gut.
- **Possible results:** Redness, acne, rosacea due to inflammation; faster formation of lines and wrinkles as hormone levels lower; skin problems, such as acne, eczema or dermatitis, that are caused by food intolerances.

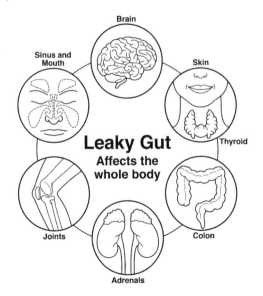

When it comes to aging, protecting the lining of the gut from damage is as important as protecting your skin externally against factors such as UV damage.

As the name suggests, leaky gut is a condition in which damage occurs to the intestinal lining. Normally the gut lining is a smooth, tubal area lined with a layer of cells that creates a protective coating for the lining underneath it. This lining houses immune cells that alert the bowel quickly to any substances trying to enter a part of the body where they don't belong. The job of the gut lining is to let out nutrients while simultaneously preventing any toxins from the bloodstream entering the bowel. It must also ensure any particles of undigested foods, viruses, bacteria or toxins on their way to be excreted from the bowel leave the system rather than being reabsorbed. As one of the largest surface areas in the human body—and one of the few places exposed to the outside world (via things we ingest)—it's not surprising that the lining of the bowel takes this job extremely seriously, carefully regulating exactly what can pass in or pass out of those holes. It's like border patrol for your body.

Particles must be very small to leave the gut—they pass out via the cells themselves or via gaps between these cells known as tight junctions. They are escorted by special carrier proteins that act like taxi drivers, ferrying them through the holes—larger particles can't attach to these proteins; it would be like an elephant trying to get into the taxi. When leaky gut develops, the tight junctions start to loosen and the spaces between the cells start to widen. The result is that toxins and larger molecules of food that normally pass out of the intestine can start to leak into the circulatory system of their own accord; they no longer need the body's taxis (special carrier proteins) to take them there. Not only does this mean food is passing out of the intestine before all the nutrients in it are being absorbed (a cause of malabsorption—see page 16), but these larger food particles also confuse your immune system. They aren't a form it has seen before and so it thinks they are there to do harm and it signals the immune system to attack them. This causes the immune cells to flood your body with those skin-damaging inflammatory substances, but in some people this reaction may even trigger food intolerances and allergies—another problem that is closely linked to skin problems and skin aging. I'll talk about these in far more detail in the next chapter because I firmly believe that what you eat, and whether it's good for your body, clearly shows up on your skin and that adjusting your diet to counteract this can very rapidly reverse some of the signs of aging. But, if you want to fight intolerances, you also need to focus on healing any signs of leaky gut.

There's no simple home test for leaky gut, so you'll need to check your symptoms to find out if it might be behind your digestive— and skin—woes. Symptoms can include regular bouts of diarrhea or constipation, and excessive gas and bloating that can make you feel as if you're eight months pregnant by the end of the day. The development of new food intolerances—or old ones being triggered even if you eat smaller amounts of the food you're sensitive to—is also a common warning sign. Check your nails: people with leaky gut rarely grow their nails past the tops of their fingertips, or they develop vertical lines and ridges on their nails.

If I suspect leaky gut in a patient I normally order a permeability test. This involves drinking a solution containing sugars not normally absorbed by the body and a few hours later giving a urine sample. If digestion is healthy, these sugars should not be found in the urine; if they are, it's a sign that your gut lining has become more permeable and that you need to take steps to help boost its integrity. I then often follow up with a stool test, which involves taking samples over three consecutive days. This analyzes the balance of bacteria in the gut and who (or what) might be living alongside them.

So why exactly does the gut lining start to fail in this way? One reason is dysbiosis—those short-chain fatty acids that the good gut bacteria produce help keep the gut lining intact. Good bacteria also help neutralize substances called bile acids, which aid digestion but can damage the gut lining if left in contact with it for too long. Gluten, a protein found in foods containing wheat, barley or rye, can also cause damage to the gut lining as it causes the release of a protein called zonulin that can break apart the tight junctions. Finally, lack of nutrients caused by poor absorption also creates a weaker gut lining, as do stress, high-sugar diets, alcohol, drugs—including commonly used medicine like non-steroidal anti-inflammatories, such as ibuprofen—and some parasites or bacteria.

Parasites, bacteria and bugs—the secret skin invaders

The word "parasites" might have surprised you there—after all, it's not something you expect to read in a book that's essentially about beauty and looking good! But parasites feed off the gut lining and cause huge instability in the gut flora that effectively creates an entourage of harmful bacteria around them. If you have a parasite in your system, there's no doubt you will age faster. And a surprising number of you reading this could be carrying one. When the Centers for Disease Control and Prevention (CDC) in Atlanta analyzed 216,275 stool samples from the healthy population back in the 1980s, 20.1 percent of them were found to be harboring a parasite.[13] The incidence is even higher in those with gut symptoms. A UK study of stool samples of people with gut problems found 31.6 percent with at least one parasite.[14] And, yes, while traveling abroad seemed to increase the risk of picking them up, I can tell you that they don't only enter your system when in foreign climes. You can also be exposed to them from eating contaminated food in any city and even meals you prepare in your own home.

There are many types of parasites and they can cause a number of symptoms within the body, but there's one in particular that I have clearly seen affect the skin. It's called *Blastocystis hominis*, and when this has been identified and then resolved in my patients, not only do their digestion problems and energy levels improve, so does their skin. They have fewer breakouts, and the texture and tone of their skin improves. The only way to know if you have a parasite is via a stool test that detects them. But be aware, parasites rarely travel alone—once one arrives it's like the White House gates are open and everyone wants a look around, so it's important that any test you choose checks for the whole variety of pathogenic organisms that can set up shop in the bowel.

Candida, for example, is another potential invader and one I'm also increasingly seeing in patients. This is an overgrowth of a fungus called *Candida albicans*, which lives naturally in most people's system. In some people, however, it starts to overdevelop and release toxins into the system that can cause a myriad of symptoms. Gut symptoms from bloating to acid reflux; skin problems such as acne, eczema and psoriasis; and health concerns such as thrush, weight gain, sugar cravings, joint pains and fungal infections such as athlete's foot are among the extremely long list of symptoms that can signify overgrowth of candida.

The most accurate way to check for candida is a blood or stool test. The blood test looks for antibodies that the body produces against the infection, while a stool test looks for the presence of the fungus itself. If you have it you must go on a special anti-candida diet, as you have to starve the fungus of everything it needs to grow; this includes all sugars, yeasts, many fruits, some vegetables and more. It's hard to know exactly what to give up without professional advice and even harder to ensure you're eating a balanced diet if you do stick to it properly. If you suspect you have candida, I would suggest getting tested before you follow the plans in this book as it's important to eradicate it before trying to do anything else to heal the gut; if it's found, it requires specialist intervention to ensure this is done correctly. I'd suggest you work with a naturopathic doctor, nutritionist or other integrative health practitioner to eradicate it. Do not try to do it alone.

Finally, there's a problem called small intestinal bacterial overgrowth (SIBO). This occurs when your gut bacteria move into a part of the bowel in which they don't generally appear. Normally, the bacteria in the bowel are located mostly in the colon. In SIBO, however, they start to populate the small intestine instead. This can lead to symptoms such as bloating, diarrhea, constipation and gut pains. Exactly what causes it isn't known, although it's been linked to low levels of stomach acid that allow the bacteria to move to places they normally can't inhabit. Another theory is that food poisoning damages the nerves of the bowel, which stops the gut from contracting effectively—bacteria then get a chance to take hold in an area they would normally pass through. Interestingly, SIBO is commonly associated with acne and rosacea.

Because the symptoms of SIBO can be very vague (many people with irritable bowel syndrome, or IBS, actually have SIBO), it's important to rule it out if it's suspected. There are breath tests for SIBO, but they don't always give accurate results, so if a doctor suspects it, the most common way to diagnose it is to try to treat it and see what happens. If your symptoms normalize, SIBO was causing them; if not, something else is behind them. The drug you'll be given to do this is called rifaximin and it's an antibiotic—obviously if you do take this it's important to work on repopulating the bowel with healthy bacteria quickly afterward, and you may need to go on a SIBO-specific diet to try to stop the problem from recurring.

What Is Rosacea?

I've already mentioned this a few times, but it's a condition you may not have heard of—or may be a little confused by. Rosacea is a skin condition characterized by redness or flushing of the facial skin. It's often accompanied by blemishes, which is why it used to be called acne rosacea, but it's not the same as acne itself. Rosacea can also make the face feel hot or sting. The exact cause has not been determined, but in my experience it's definitely linked to food intolerances and imbalanced gut bacteria, which leads to high levels of inflammation and leaky gut. Attacks can be triggered by factors including alcohol consumption, spicy foods, sunlight and hot drinks. In my experience, healing the gut can play a huge role in reducing the look of rosacea and the number of flare-ups patients experience.

Love Your Liver

When the gut barrier fails, toxins that normally pass out of the bowel as waste can instead head back into circulation. At this point the load on the liver also increases. When it comes to hardworking organs in the body, the liver needs some kind of award. It has over 500 different jobs to do each day. It stores nutrients such as iron and vitamin B12 for when you need them, and it detoxifies the hundreds, if not thousands, of chemicals that we're exposed to every single day. If you then start adding to that load with toxins that it already thinks it's handled, it's not surprising the liver can become overloaded.

At this point it can't cope with everything coming in, which then causes a "queue" of toxins waiting to be tackled—and some of those toxins don't like to wait. Think of it as joining a long line outside a restaurant: if the line doesn't move, some people will leave and go and do something else and return later—that's exactly what happens with the toxins. They leave and recirculate in the body, but the problem is that as they travel around the bloodstream they bind on to protein molecules and change their structure. This makes them even more toxic than they were in their original state and even harder for the liver to process when they do finally make their way back there. These toxins can directly impact the skin, causing acne and faster aging, but the liver is also the organ concerned with processing hormones through the system. If it's not working effectively, you end up with hormonal imbalances that can age the body in many ways. If you want to age well, you want a liver that's performing well.

PROBLEM 4: POOR ELIMINATION

- **Why it causes aging:** Toxins not passed out via the bowel get rediverted through the skin. As they travel through the skin's layers, they can cause direct damage to collagen and elastin fibers.
- **Possible results:** Sallow complexion; adult acne; faster collagen breakdown.

A healthy bowel is reflected in the look of the skin. If the bowel is stagnated, the skin will suffer and look as congested as your insides. Remember: if you go, you glow.

The last part of the digestive process is elimination. When we visit the bathroom to defecate we pass out a mixture of undigested food, natural waste by-products, such as cells and bacteria, and some of the toxins we encounter each day. Clearing your system of these things is key to a clean, well-functioning body and good skin.

If you're not going to the bathroom as often as you should, or your bowel isn't moving things through quite as quickly as it should, food starts to sit for longer in the intestine. At this point it starts to ferment. Not only does this create a tasty food source for the types of bacteria you don't want in your body, it also puts pressure on the gut wall, which can contribute to leaky gut. But, more importantly, as food hangs around the bowel, toxins and hormones that are supposed to be leaving the body get a second chance to re-enter the system—especially if the gut wall is leaking. This can cause hormonal imbalances—which, as I'll explain in Chapter 4, can speed up aging—but also lead to less than healthy-looking skin. Why? Because if toxins can't leave the bowel via excretion, the body will attempt to eliminate them via the other detoxifying organs—one of which is the skin. The most common manifestation of this is a sallow-looking skin prone to acne and breakouts, but as toxins pass up through the structural layers of skin they can also damage collagen and elastin fibers, leading to a loss of firmness and the development of fine lines and wrinkles.

So, are you eliminating poorly? Well, sometimes I ask a patient how many bowel movements they have in a day, and they look surprised and say, "A day? I only go twice a week." While it's defined as normal to go to the bathroom anything from three times a day to three times a week, I don't want you to be normal—I want you to be the healthiest you can be and I believe it's optimum to go once a day as that ensures waste is regularly leaving the body.

So what should you be aiming for when you do go? At the most basic, you should go to the bathroom once a day and it should be an easy process; but, if you really want to get into details, there is actually a blueprint for a perfect poop, and this is it:

- It should be medium to light brown (some medications or supplements might alter this, but, generally, brown is good).
- It should be easy to pass without straining.
- It should be formed into one stool—not lots of small pieces.
- It should also be smooth—not covered in cracks and lines.
- It should be S-shaped, as that reflects the shape of the intestine.
- It should gently slide into the water, not land with a big cannonball-like splash that leaves your butt damp! Once in the bowl, it should sink slowly.
- It's okay if there's a smell, but it shouldn't be too strong.

If these bullet points aren't all true, then something about your digestive health could be improved. If you're getting obvious bowel symptoms, such as bloating, gas, loose stools or constipation, it's likely at least one of them apply.

Poor elimination can be improved by boosting overall gut health, but other ways to improve things include drinking more water, as hydration makes stools easier to pass, and including more of the gentler types of fiber in your diet. This is called insoluble fiber, and it's found in many fruits, vegetables, quinoa, rice and potatoes. If you need some extra help, drinks or powders containing psyllium fiber can also help move things along until you get your digestion working effectively again.

THE WHOLE PICTURE

I'm aware that's been a lot to take in, but I hope you can now clearly see how an unhealthy gut can fundamentally influence many of the processes involved with aging. If not, perhaps this illustration might make things clearer—sometimes it's just easier to show things in pictures.

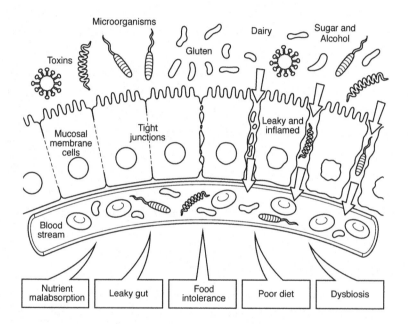

But before I explain how you can change things, there's something very important I need to mention.

THINGS TO RULE OUT

While in most of the patients I see, one, or a combination, of the aforementioned problems is the cause of their gut issues, there are also some more serious or complicated conditions that can manifest in gut symptoms. These must be ruled out before you start a home treatment plan.

Celiac disease

This condition is caused when the immune system reacts to the gluten that is found in foods containing wheat, rye and barley, or to a similar protein found in oats. With celiac disease there are gastrointestinal symptoms, such as bloating, abdominal pain and erratic bowel movements. It's extremely common, affecting 1 in 100 people in the US and the UK, but not everyone with it has been diagnosed. In the UK alone, it's estimated that half a million people with celiac disease have no idea they are affected.[15] In the US it's believed there could be 1.4 million undiagnosed sufferers.[16]

Celiac disease is diagnosed via a blood test that shows the presence of antibodies to gluten in the system. If the result is positive, a second test is normally done, which takes a biopsy of the bowel to look at tiny finger-like projections called villi within it. These flatten in celiac disease and the sight of this confirms the diagnosis suggested by the blood test. It's very important that you are still eating food with gluten at the time of the test or it won't give accurate results. If you are found to have celiac disease, you will have to go on a gluten-free diet for the rest of your life.

Bile acid diarrhea (BAD)

If severe diarrhea is the main symptom of your tummy woes, you should ask your doctor about BAD. Causing very frequent watery stools, sufferers can need the bathroom up to 10 times a day. It's caused by higher than normal levels of bile acids (produced by the liver as part of the digestive process) reaching the colon, which speeds up gut transit time triggering frequent stools. It can be diagnosed via a test called a SeHCAT scan, but carrying this out requires swallowing a trackable chemical that's scanned as it passes through your body, so it's a complicated, expensive test that isn't offered everywhere. A much cheaper diagnostic tool, therefore, is to give suspected sufferers a drug called cholestyramine. This binds to any excess bile acid and stops the symptoms. If it's diagnosed your doctor will suggest you stay on cholestyramine.

Inflammatory bowel disease or cancers

Only a very small percentage of people that I see have digestive problems caused by inflammatory bowel disease or cancers, but you should be aware of the possibility. Problems such as colitis, Crohn's disease and some cancers can manifest with gut symptoms. If your gut woes come associated with any of the following, it's important to see your doctor before you start on the plans in this book, just to rule out any more serious underlying conditions:

- If your symptoms came on very suddenly; if you see blood in your stools or you start to lose weight for no obvious reason.
- If you suffer heartburn or acid reflux more than three times a week for weeks at a time, or have trouble swallowing or hoarseness of the voice.
- If any bloating you suffer doesn't come and go through the day but instead leaves you with a permanently distended stomach—and you are also suffering from feelings of fullness when you eat very little and before you would usually feel full, and/or abdominal pain.

THE GUT-BALANCING CCP PLAN

Healing the gut is absolutely the most fundamental step to fight premature aging, and it needs to be well underway before you start any of the other plans that follow. Because it is so important, I suggest you follow the tips below for four weeks at the very least, but ideally two or three months, before you start integrating the advice from the chapters that follow. That may sound like a long time, but Rome wasn't built in a day and, in body terms, your gut is more akin to a universe than a city like Rome! It will take time to bring it back into balance, and the higher your level of digest-aging, the longer it is going to take. I know that might sound frustrating, particularly in a world where we are used to quick-fix promises and immediate gratification, but it could have taken many years for your body to reach the level of digest-aging that you are affected by, so it will take more than the blink of an eye to reverse that.

The good news is that the skin is a very responsive organ. It regenerates roughly every 28 days—as such, you will start to see a difference in its look and feel quite quickly, and I'm hoping that will keep you motivated to keep up the good work for as long as it takes to restore optimum health inside as well.

This Gut-Balancing CCP Plan has three specific stages—Clear, Correct and Protect—which follows established naturopathic healing principles. Again, it's important to follow them in this order. This will ensure you get optimum results and will also keep you from spending money on supplements such as probiotics that can't repopulate the bowel if the gut hasn't at least started to heal and rebuild, or vitamin supplements, which can't be absorbed because you don't have the right balance of gut bacteria to help with that task; both just lead to expensive urine.

As for how long you should spend doing each section, I would suggest a 2:1:1 ratio—so, for example, spend two weeks on the steps in the Clear plan, keep those up and add in the steps from the Correct part of the plan for one week, then also add in those from the Protect section for the fourth week. If you feel your gut needs some extra help, then continue the plan at this point for two to three months until everything completely stabilizes.

You will also notice sections called "Power Up." These aren't essential for everyone, but if you do have a lot of symptoms and a high level of digest-aging, I would strongly suggest that you consider following them. A lot of the suggestions here involve supplements, but please do not take any without discussing with your doctor, particularly if you are on any other medication, using herbal remedies or if you could be pregnant.

Clear

The first step in making over your gut is to remove anything doing it harm—you can't try to fix something that's continuously being attacked. There are three main things you should consider here:

1) Eliminate the main gut damagers

There are so many of these it can seem a daunting task, but here are some of the things that you need to eliminate from your diet and lifestyle—or at least avoid as much as possible—while you try to heal the gut.

- **The Ultimate Agers:** Four foods are going to come up time and time again within this book as foods that harm the body and increase the rate as which you age. These are gluten, dairy, sugar and alcohol. If you want to reverse the signs of aging, if you want a healthy gut, if you want to fight inflammation, if you simply want to thrive, I urge you to eliminate these foods from your diet. I'm aware that isn't easy, but before you throw your hands up in horror and wonder what on earth you're going to eat if you do that, following the Age-Reversing Eating Plan starting on page 204 will automatically cut all of these out for you for 28 days, making things simple. If you do decide your body thrives without one or more of them, you'll find lots of advice in Chapter 2 (where I discuss exactly how these foods impact your health and the way your skin looks and behaves) on how to replace them.
- **Medicines:** I'm not saying never take another drug, but if you're regularly taking non-steroidal anti-inflammatory drugs (NSAIDs), such as aspirin or ibuprofen, for headaches or back pain, it would be better to try to find the root cause of that pain and tackle that rather than simply masking the symptoms. When pain does strike, you might also like to try some natural alternatives to help combat it—these might include:
  - » **Acupuncture:** This can help many pain-related conditions, including back pain and headaches. I have been able to help many patients with acupuncture and seen them come off NSAIDs after using it.
  - » **Arnica:** This is a homeopathic remedy and can be used in the form of tablets, creams, ointments or as a tincture. It comes from the arnica plant and it's particularly good for fighting the pain of sprains, strains, and muscle and joint pain. It also helps with bruising.

» **Boswellia:** Made from tree resin, this is a natural anti-inflammatory. It's also particularly effective in helping to reduce arthritis pain.

» **Devil's claw:** This herbal remedy is licensed to tackle back pain and is available in health food stores or drug stores. It helps fight inflammation. Take it as directed on the pack.

» **Tiger Balm or menthol-based pain relief sticks and gels:** Applied to the skin, these create sensations of heat that actually interrupt the body's pain signals. They work particularly well for headaches. Simply apply them to the back of the neck or forehead.

Also, limit antibiotics. Many of us take them when they aren't needed—coughs and colds are a classic example of this. Antibiotics only attack bacteria, but colds are caused by viruses, so they will make absolutely no difference to how your symptoms progress, yet every winter thousands of people ask their doctors for them. The good news is, the growing threat of antibiotic resistance means doctors are becoming more reluctant to give antibiotics unless they are strictly necessary, so listen to their advice and only use them when they are essential for tackling infection.

• **Stress:** It's important to try to manage this. Chronic stress is extremely damaging to the entire body, including the gut and the skin. It's also a major trigger for inflammation; I'll talk more about ways to manage stress in Chapter 6.

• **Foods that trigger intolerances or allergies**: Finding these and eliminating them will help boost body health. The Age-Reversing Eating Plan avoids the five main problem foods that I see in my clinic—these are slightly different to the four Ultimate Agers I mentioned on page 39. However, as it's possible to be intolerant to any food (I'll tell you about the surprising one I react to later), it's important that you have an idea of how to spot what might be causing problems. I'll discuss some ways to do this in the next chapter.

POWER UP

Consider having a stool test to help identify any hitchhiking parasites in your system. If you use a good laboratory, it can also give you a detailed profile of exactly what's going on within your bowel. It can analyze, for example, the type of bacteria you have in your system, helping you determine if dysbiosis is present. It can also look at how well you are digesting or absorbing nutrients and may pinpoint a food allergy (although it won't be able to say exactly what it's to). You can work with a naturopathic doctor, or other integrative physician, to organize your testing. If the test comes up positive, you will need professional help to remove any "hitchhikers" from your body.

2) Go organic whenever possible

This reduces your exposure to chemicals such as pesticides that can stress the gut and the liver. Eat pesticides and it's like New Year's Eve for the bad bacteria in your gut. Ideally I'd want everything you eat to be organic, but I know it's more expensive and that this isn't possible for everyone, so at the very least try to follow these rules:

- Choose organic versions of the foods you eat most in your diet—if you're consuming something daily, try to swap to an organic version.
- Most pesticides collect in the skin of a fruit or vegetable, so it's less important to choose organic versions of produce where you don't consume the skin, such as oranges, melons, bananas and avocados, and more important for foods such as grapes, tomatoes and berries, where you do eat the skin.
- Chop the tops off root vegetables, such as carrots or rutabegas, as this is where most pesticide exposure occurs. For the same reason, remove the outer leaves of foods such as cabbages.

- When you're eating meat or poultry, choose grass-fed or free-range versions and remove any visible fat, as this is where pollutants collect.
- Wash and, where appropriate, scrub with a small brush all produce for 20–30 seconds before you eat it.

Correct

Once you've removed the things that might be disrupting the bowel, it's time to replace things that you might be lacking.

1) Take a probiotic supplement

These help restore levels of good bacteria to the system. Different strains improve health in different ways. To improve general digestive health, though, I recommend a probiotic that contains the DDS-1 strain of *Lactobacillus acidophilus* and *Bifidobacterium lactis*. This is the most proven probiotic in regards to quality, stability and clinical relevance. I've also created my own probiotic called Healthy Flora that has this strain mixed with an antioxidant called grapeseed extract—a combination that gives the skin and gut a glow from the inside out. You can find Healthy Flora at www.drnigma.com and www.net-a-porter.com.

2) Increase your fiber levels

Fiber helps the gut in a number of ways. It is an essential food for the good bacteria and the substance from which they produce those important short-chain fatty acids. It also helps bulk out stools, making them easier to pass and ensuring that your system is more regular. Not surprisingly, the first thing many people will do if they are experiencing gut symptoms is to add more fiber to their diet, but some of them are then rather surprised to find that any digestive problems they are suffering from actually worsen.

The reason for this is that if you add fiber before the gut is ready, it won't digest effectively; it will ferment and you will bloat. As we've already discussed, that could potentially feed the bad bacteria and damage the gut lining further. However, once the gut has begun its natural healing process, fibrous foods will be more likely to have those positive benefits you expected. Foods containing soluble fiber, such as rice, quinoa, potatoes, banana and papaya, are gentler on the gut. Insoluble fiber (in foods such as bran, seeds, nuts and beans) is a little rougher. If you still find fiber upsets you, try focusing on soluble forms of fiber.

3) Balance your stomach acid levels

If you tried the baking soda test (see page 20) and discovered you are prone to low acid levels, then chewing for longer is absolutely the first change you need to make in your eating regimen. Eat sitting a table, take time over meals, ensure each mouthful is chewed to the consistency of a smooth paste before you swallow it and take a break between mouthfuls. If that doesn't seem to help, try stimulating your levels of stomach acid before meals.

One simple way to do this is to have a first course containing some bitter leaves, such as arugula or radicchio, which stimulate the digestive juices. You could also try drinking a quarter teaspoon of apple cider vinegar or some digestive bitters in water about 10–15 minutes before meals containing protein. Try not to drink it with your meals, though, as this can also dilute acid levels.

POWER UP

If problems don't resolve naturally with those simple changes, you might want to try a supplement containing Betaine HCl, a form of hydrochloric acid. The best ones also supply the enzyme pepsin to more naturally mimic the stomach's environment.

You do have to be a little careful when taking acid supplements because if you don't have low acid they can actually cause more problems than they solve. The rules for using them are as follows:

- Don't use them if you are regularly using anti-inflammatory drugs, such as ibuprofen, or if you have any damage to the gastric tract, such as an ulcer.

- Stomach acid is involved in the digestion of protein-based foods. If you are not eating protein in that meal you do not need to supplement and shouldn't take them.

- If you feel your stomach burning after taking the supplement, you do not have low stomach acid levels and don't need to supplement.

4) Boost your digestive enzymes

Again, enzyme production can also be increased if you chew your food well and take time over your meals. This allows the brain to send the signals to the stomach that get things moving. Eating small meals also helps ensure you don't overwhelm your system with more food than it can comfortably handle.

POWER UP

If this doesn't improve your symptoms, you may want to supplement with digestive enzymes. Choose a formula that contains all of the three enzymes you need—amylase, protease and lipase. Some supplements use animal-based sources of these, but if you are vegetarian, look for formulas containing papain, which digests protein, and bromelain, which helps you digest both protein and fat. As with acid supplements, see a health professional before taking these if you have any damage to the gut.

Protect

The final step is to treat the gut in ways that actively promote restoration and repair. You want to heal the gut, not just mask all the symptoms you've been experiencing up until now.

1) Eat mucosa-boosting foods

There are many foods that can help rebuild the mucus layer that protects the gut, and adding them regularly to your daily diet, if you don't eat them already, can rebuild and repair the gut lining. Good examples include cabbage, which is rich in the antioxidant glutamine; bone broths, which are extremely healing (see recipe on page 239); and fermented foods and drinks, such as sauerkraut, kimchi, miso, tempeh and kombucha. Many of these are readily available in most supermarkets now, or you can buy them online at specialty foods stores. Also add plenty of foods to your diet that contain vitamin A and zinc, as these are the nutrients your body needs to support the integrity of all mucous membranes. These include yellow, red and orange fruits and vegetables, such as carrots, sweet potatoes, apricots and butternut squash (while these don't contain vitamin A per se, your body converts a substance they do contain, betacarotene, into vitamin A), leafy green vegetables, red meat, lentils, shellfish and seeds, such as pumpkin or sesame.

2) Add some prebiotics

You have already started to replenish your levels of gut bacteria by taking a probiotic supplement, but your final step in trying to create a healthy microbiome is feeding those bacteria so they start to reproduce and repopulate. The foods that do this are called prebiotics. They include the fermented foods described above, but foods that contain the fiber inulin are also excellent prebiotics—these include sweet potatoes, yams, leeks, garlic, onions and Jerusalem artichokes. Have three portions of these a week to provide the fuel your gut bacteria need.

POWER UP

Take deglycyrrhizinated licorice (DGL): when it comes to healing the gut, this is just amazing. The recommended dose is one to three tablets a day, and each tablet should contain 380–400 mg of DGL. This is not the same as the licorice you find in candy stores, or the tea from herbal stores. These are made from licorice root that contains a substance called glycyrrhizin. Glycyrrhizin is contraindicated in people with high blood pressure, but DGL has had this removed—and a good brand should state on the label that it contains less than 1–2 percent glycyrrhizin. Despite this, if you do have high blood pressure, please see your doctor before taking DGL.

Also try taking mastic gum, which works very well alongside DGL. It's made on an island off Greece from tree resin and it was originally used to treat ulcers, but it also helps repair the gut mucosa all the way from the esophagus to the rectum. It can also help fight *Helicobacter pylori*, a bacteria that can live in the stomach and which has been linked to the formation of ulcers and may also trigger symptoms of acid reflux. Try taking 1,000 mg once or twice a day (depending on the severity of your symptoms) for two months.

While this combination is the thing I will include in every gut repair program, you might also like to think about drinking a dose of aloe vera juice daily, which helps with gut repair, and/or taking a supplement of the amino acid glutamine. This has been shown in many studies to help repair the intestinal lining and help increase nutrient uptake. The dose for glutamine is 1,000–1,500 mg daily. Slippery elm is another supplement I use. It's an appropriate name as it makes a slippery gel when mixed with water. I use this all the time to heal the gut as it contains mucilage, which your body naturally produces to protect the gut lining, but it also stimulates nerve endings in the intestinal tract, which encourage it to repair itself. Use 400-500 mg, three to four times daily for four to eight weeks.

So, that's it: you now have the key information about how digestion affects aging; we've covered everything you need to know about the gut itself and how the problems within it might be affecting your skin. As part of this, I've touched on how what you eat affects the gut, but now let's look a little more closely at how specific foods can have an impact.

CHAPTER 2

EATING BEAUTY

You are what you eat. This is what I say to each and every one of my patients because I've observed it in thousands of them over the years—whatever you put into your body will show up on your skin. Food can be your skin's medicine, but it can also be a poison. It can heal the skin, or wreak havoc upon it. I have seen eating the wrong diet create premature aging on someone's skin in a very short period of time. In fact, it's now gotten to the point where someone can walk into my clinic and I can see immediately in their face if they have a sensitivity to, or are consuming too much of, some foods or drinks. Time and time again the same signs show up on the face. I call it the Four Faces of Aging.

Don't think that it takes years for those changes to manifest; with some foods it can take as little as a weekend of overdoing it for your skin to develop signs such as acne, puffiness, changes in skin tone, premature fine lines and wrinkles, sagging, loss of luster, or dark circles under the eyes. If you already have these problems genetically, they'll be worsened by eating the wrong types of foods for you—what's healthy for one person might be inflammatory for another.

This is why determining what those wrong foods might be is tricky. People are so confused about what to eat—and I'm not surprised. One diet says eat fewer carbohydrates, another says eat only carbohydrates; one says fast, the other says graze all day … I wish I could make it easier for you, but the truth is I don't believe there is a one-size-fits-all medicine, nor is there a one-size-fits-all diet. Each person might require something a little different, depending on their level of a state I refer to as gut-flammation.

Gut-flammation is like a fire burning inside the gut, damaging everything it touches. It occurs as a result of all the problems we discussed in the last chapter—increased dysbiosis, damage to the gut lining, increased intestinal permeability and the vicious circle of damage this then sets off—but what you're eating day by day can also contribute to its development, as you're about to discover.

HOW TO USE THIS CHAPTER

This chapter differs from the last one in that it doesn't have a specific plan for everyone to follow—instead the advice within it should be used to pinpoint changes that might create the most benefits for you personally. Use it to analyze what your symptoms might be saying about how your body reacts to the foods you eat, and use that information to help keep you focused as you follow the Gut-Balancing CCP Plan on page 37. There's lots of advice in this chapter that explains how to make following that plan easier. For example, I explore how to replace staple foods such as bread and pasta in your diet, which can seem quite overwhelming when you first start. Also, use this chapter to potentially think long term. The negative changes you see in your skin are signs that your body is out of balance and perhaps, once you're more aware of your trigger foods, you may want to cut back on, or even completely eliminate, them forever.

WHEN GOOD FOODS GO BAD

Estimates suggest almost 50 percent of the population suffer some form of reaction to one or more of the foods they eat and many people have absolutely no idea it's happening. Hidden food allergies or intolerances can manifest within 10 minutes after eating a food, or symptoms may take as long as 3 days to occur. While some patients are really in tune with their bodies and can spot foods that cause problems quickly, others have no idea that something they might eat every single day could be the cause of their skin—and health—woes.

As such, many of my patients are shocked when I test them for intolerances and they come up positive. They are equally surprised that once they avoid these foods, skin problems such as eczema, under-eye bags, red, blotchy cheeks and even lines and wrinkles resolve in as little as a month, as well as other problems, such as weight gain, headaches, joint pains, bloating and gas that they may have had for years. It is mind-boggling that dermatologists and primary care physicians rarely look at what their patients are eating and how the gut is reacting as part of diagnosing health issues.

When it comes to allergies and intolerances, there's a lot of confusion out there, not least because people often interchange the terms. Here's how to tell them apart:

Food allergies

These can range from mild skin rashes to life-threatening anaphylactic shock and occur when the immune system reacts to a food you consume. Allergic reactions happen extremely quickly after eating a food and it's unlikely that by adulthood someone with a true food allergy doesn't know exactly what food they are allergic to. While it's possible to be allergic to any food, the most common food-related allergies are to peanuts, eggs, milk, seeds, shellfish and citrus fruit. About 1–2 percent of the population have this type of allergy.

Food intolerances or sensitivities

With an intolerance or sensitivity, the body reacts to a food but it's a far slower reaction, taking potentially 72 hours to show symptoms, and those symptoms can be much more insidious. Food intolerance can manifest in almost every part of the body from top (headaches and migraines) to toe (some experts even believe bunions can be aggravated by intolerances to dairy). Because of this, many people with food sensitivities have no idea they have one and often think symptoms such as loose bowel movements or a permanently runny nose are normal because they have never really known anything different. The other difference between intolerances and allergies is exactly which immune cells are involved in the reaction. True allergies trigger a rapid response from a type of antibody called IgE; with intolerances, however, the immune system marshals a different set of antibodies known as IgG, which react more slowly—this causes some experts to refer to intolerances now as delayed allergy syndrome. Think of it this way—E comes before G in the alphabet and E reactions also appear before G ones. Exact figures for IgG reactions are hard to come by, but some estimates suggest that 45–60 percent of the population could be intolerant to at least one food or more.

In this book we'll mostly be focusing on IgG intolerances because people with true allergies tend to be aware of them and avoid the foods that cause them problems, and because IgG reactions are the ones I see so commonly affecting skin and causing premature aging.

What Are Free Radicals?
Your body produces thousands of free radicals every day; very simply, they are molecules that have an odd number of electrons. Normally electrons appear in pairs and so when a free radical forms, it basically tries to snatch its missing electron from molecules around it. That molecule then ends up with an unpaired electron of its own, which it then tries to match—so it then starts to repeat the process. This constant chopping and changing eventually damages the cell. You may have heard that antioxidants fight free radical damage. The reason is that they donate an electron to any unpaired molecules, which stops them from having to steal them from those within your cells.

There are a few different reasons why this occurs. An IgG reaction causes inflammation, the enemy that I'll discuss at length in the next chapter. When your immune system starts to react against a food to which it is sensitive, it triggers the release of inflammatory chemicals that impact every part of the body, including the skin. The inflammation caused by food intolerances can cause or worsen acne. It can also cause pigmentation changes, bloating, puffiness and under-eye bags, redness and a blotchy skin tone that all add years to a face—and that's the damage you can see. Inflammation also weakens the skin's barrier, leaving it susceptible to free radical damage, which degrades collagen and elastin.

The body also finds intolerance reactions stressful, and this causes the release of the stress hormone cortisol, which also impacts on skin. Cortisol can damage collagen (see page 148), and it slows its rate of repair. It also decreases the skin's ability to synthesize a vital molecule called hyaluronic acid. This helps pull moisture into the skin and helps it retain a plump, youthful texture. Cortisol also thins the upper layers of the skin and makes the blood vessels underneath more prominent, creating a blotchy, red complexion that adds years (in a study by the Ludwig-Boltzmann-Institute for Urban Ethology in Austria[1], it was found that uneven skin tone could add 20 years to how old people thought a face looked). Another response that occurs in the body during an intolerance reaction is a rise in insulin levels and sugars, and, as you'll see shortly, sugar is the worst food for directly aging the skin. If there are high levels of sugar in your bloodstream, you will age faster—in fact, studies show that people with type 2 diabetes (who commonly have high blood-sugar levels) have levels of aging compounds in their skin three times higher than those in the general population.[2]

Eliminating IgG reactive foods from your diet can improve not only your skin but help resolve long-term issues that you might not even realize are food related—migraines, headaches, IBS, bloating and chronic fatigue, for example. This too can make you look younger. Think about it: if you have niggling health problems that cause you discomfort or worry, it's going to show in your facial expressions. You'll hold tension in your forehead and between your brows, creating frown lines. When your health problems start to resolve and the tension disappears, your face will relax, softening those lines as it does so. You'll feel better, and as a consequence of that, you'll start to look better.

The interesting thing about food intolerances is that they can be triggered by any food—even those that enter your diet in the smallest quantities. I'm intolerant to garlic—if I eat garlic, it triggers a clear inflammatory reaction in my body. It puts my gut completely out—I get a bit of joint pain, an upset tummy and I'll always, always, get a zit on my face—to me it's a clear sign that that food doesn't agree with my body. This proves that literally anything could be a trigger food, but, saying that, there are five foods that come up time and time again when I test people for intolerances in the clinic, and so I always suggest people look at these before they start analyzing every food they consume. They are:

- **Cow's milk dairy:** While it's moderately tolerated by some people, a lot of people find they react to dairy. In fact, there are at least four different substances in milk that people react to, including lactose, casein, a protein called A1 and whey. You can have a problem with one of these substances or a combination of them.
- **Gluten:** I talk about gluten over and over again because it's so important. There are three different types of reactions that can occur in response to gluten—celiac disease (see page 36), a problem called non-celiac gluten sensitivity and general intolerance.
- **Soy:** I have mixed feelings about soy. It can have beneficial effects on hormone levels in the body but there's no doubt that many patients react to it. The main thing to remember is that not all soy is created equally. Genetically modified soy or processed soy, such as that in soy milk, might be more likely to cause reactions and damage the gut than fermented soy, the type that is traditionally eaten in Asia. If you want to include soy products in your diet, choose forms such as tempeh, miso, natto or Korean pastes, such as doenjang, over the more processed products.

- **Eggs:** Eggs are a very common problem food, and what I'm seeing now is that people who have egg intolerance are also developing problems eating chicken, possibly due to a cross-reaction with something in the feed the birds are eating.
- **Yeast:** I see issues with yeast in so many patients with gut problems. There are two types of yeast that most commonly appear in our food today—baker's yeast and brewer's yeast—and they can appear in more than the obvious bread and beer you'd expect them in. Yeast-containing products can also include croissants, doughnuts, muffins, wine, cider, stock cubes and gravies, and yeast spreads such as Vegemite. Many condiments, particularly those that use vinegar, can contain yeast, as can some vitamin B supplements.

DISCOVERING FOOD INTOLERANCE

There are two ways to discover a food intolerance: follow an elimination diet or, as I recommend to most of my patients, have a blood test.

The elimination diet

Let's start with the elimination diet. This is an attempt to figure out which foods are causing gut-flammation by keeping a food diary (see page 56). You remove the suspect foods completely from your diet for three weeks. If your symptoms disappear during that time, it's extremely likely that one of the foods you removed is causing your problems. You then use a little trial and error to try to find out which food it is by introducing the foods again, one by one. Try eating a portion of the food, alone, ideally on an empty stomach, then wait 72 hours to see if any symptoms return. Remember, it could take anything from 20 minutes to 3 days for anything to happen, but because you're not used to the food, chances are your body will mount a reaction quite quickly and give you a clear sign if it's a problem food for you.

If you don't notice any symptoms reappearing within 72 hours, that is not a food to which you're intolerant and you can add it back into your diet. Now repeat the process with your next suspect food. Keep repeating until you find the culprit. If nothing shows up, then it could be something completely different that's causing your problem (some people, for example, might suspect they can't eat potatoes, but, actually, they always add vinegar to their fries and it's the vinegar that they react to)! This is why spotting intolerances can be so hard to do on your own and why it's better to work with a naturopathic doctor or nutritionist if you can; if that isn't possible, though, use my blueprint on how to write a good food diary (page 56), which can help you spot patterns a bit more clearly.

An elimination diet can be a very effective method of spotting intolerances, but it does require being especially in touch with your body and following the instructions as closely as possible. It can also be hard to spot intolerances to foods that are in almost everything you eat, such as gluten or particular additives, but listen carefully and your body will tell you the truth.

A blood test

If I'm trying to diagnose an intolerance, I'll often use a blood test that checks for IgG antibodies in the system. This gives a good starting point for people who may have complex reactions or simply don't have time to use a food diary. The test I use is called the Alletess Laboratory IgG test, and it requires drawing a small sample of blood with a needle. Other tests are available that just require a finger prick, which companies then check against a number of different food allergens. The best tests check a good range of foods, but also check for different types of antibodies—this is called total IgG testing.

Most conventional doctors and specialists do not have a lot of clinical experience with IgG testing and rarely use it. They also often criticize it, and I admit it isn't perfect—it can sometimes give false negatives (where a food is given the all-clear when actually there is a problem with it), particularly if someone hasn't eaten a food for a while. However, I have never known it to give a false positive. In my clinical experience, if it says someone is intolerant to a food, then taking it out of their diet will improve their health.

Exactly how many foods someone reacts to depends on their personal level of gut-flammation, as the more problems you have with your digestion, the more likely it is that you will start to develop multiple intolerances. That's why if I find someone with a lot of reactive foods, I definitely look further into the health of their gut, even if they haven't come to see me with any obvious gut-related symptoms. Remember, health and aging start in the gut, and healing the gut can help solve more health problems than you would ever suspect.

How to Keep a Good Food Diary

Trying to spot intolerance isn't always easy. While some, such as lactose intolerance, make themselves known quite quickly (sufferers usually need to rush to the bathroom soon after eating dairy), most intolerances hide very well and you'll need to tease out the signs that show you what's behind them. Keeping a good food diary is therefore extremely important.

Date	Time	Food eaten	Ingredients	Symptoms	Time

The table above gives you an idea of what you need to record, but here are some important things to remember when you're doing it:

- Fill the diary in as you eat so that you don't forget anything.

- Write down everything you consume, including condiments and spices—and don't forget sweets, vitamins, pills, chewing gum or anything you sneak from the plates of your children or partner.
- If you are eating a processed food, write down the brand name and ingredients (or photograph the label and keep it on your phone). It might be a single preservative that causes problems, which you'll only spot if you know exactly what is in each food.
- Don't forget drinks—you can be intolerant to them too.

After a while you'll hopefully start to see patterns form. For example, you always get a headache around 3 p.m. on a Wednesday following a work meeting on Tuesday lunchtime where sandwiches are provided. If that's the only day you eat bread, then perhaps something in bread is a trigger food for you. Similarly, you get a runny nose on a Sunday morning—and Friday night is always white wine night. Things can be a little harder when it's foods you eat every day that are causing your problems as your symptoms might be more or less constant. In that case, it's when the problems don't appear that might give you a clue to their cause; what didn't you eat in the preceeding days? If you are getting stuck identifying any clear patterns, then seeking professional advice might help you spot things you can't see. Or, you may want to try IgG testing to find your answer.

Interestingly, it's often foods you crave that are the cause of intolerances. They release opiates into the brain as part of the immune response when you eat them. If you get really strong cravings for any particular foods or tastes, see if any symptom might be particularly associated with these.

Signs and symptoms of food intolerance

These are some of the most common ways a food intolerance might present itself. Remember, these can occur up to 72 hours after a trigger food, so you'll have to study your food diary clearly to try to spot patterns:

Gut symptoms
- Bloating
- Constipation
- Cramps or abdominal pain
- Diarrhea
- Gas

Health symptoms
- Cough
- Foggy thinking
- Headaches
- Itchy eyes or mouth
- Joint pains
- Low energy
- Migraines
- Mood swings
- Runny or stuffed-up nose
- Sneezing
- Weight gain
- Wheezing

Skin symptoms
- Breakouts
- Dark circles
- Dermatitis
- Eczema
- Facial puffiness
- Pigmentation
- Premature aging
- Rashes
- Under-eye bags

INTOLERANCE—THE 21ST-CENTURY EPIDEMIC

One comment I regularly hear regarding food intolerance is that our grandparents didn't suffer from them; that they didn't exist in the 1940s, '50s or '60s, and so they must be a made-up modern affliction. At least part of that statement is true. People in the past didn't seem to get the same issues with foods as we do. In fact, when researchers at the Mayo Clinic tested stored blood samples taken from Air Force recruits in the 1950s, they found over four times fewer markers for the incidence of celiac disease than they would expect to find in modern samples[3]—but that doesn't mean intolerances don't exist now. We now recognize food intolerances that our grandparents didn't, so they possibly lived with problems we might now seek help for. But it's also true that life has changed since our grandparents' time and we're now living in a world that makes the development of allergies and intolerances far more likely.

Our diet isn't the same as it used to be. Our grandparents cooked most of their food from scratch and food wasn't as chemically treated—they simply weren't exposed to the levels of added gluten, pesticides and preservatives that cause the gut damage that triggers intolerances. They also consumed less gut-damaging alcohol and sugar than we do. Their staple diet was also less wheat focused—while they may have had toast for breakfast and perhaps a sandwich for lunch, dinner was often meat, potatoes and vegetables. Snacking wasn't common either.

Contemporary food-processing methods have also changed our food. Modern wheat is farmed in ways that increase levels of the specific proteins in gluten that people react to (in fact, a 2013 Italian study, which gave celiac sufferers an ancient form of wheat called *Triticum monococcum,* found they were less likely to react to this than modern wheat).[4] In the UK, milk used to be farmed mostly from Jersey cows, which are less likely genetically to make a type of protein called A1. This protein releases a peptide into the system that can cause digestion issues in some people. Over the years, however, fewer dairy herds use Jersey cows and most milk now contains A1 protein. Milk in the US too has changed; cross-breeding with cows carrying the A1 gene has made the majority of cows in America produce milk with the A1 protein. Research at Australia's Curtin University has recently shown that going back to drinking milk that doesn't contain A1 reduced problems such as loose bowel movements, bloating and stomach cramps in many people who had problems digesting milk.[5]

Finally, life wasn't as fast paced—our grandparents usually ate at the table, not standing up while rushing to their next appointment, and this less hurried way of eating ensured they had better digestion. As I briefly mentioned before, life wasn't so clean. Our immune system was kept busy dealing with true threats such as mold in our food, bugs we picked up on our hands doing tasks more manually or playing outside when we were children, and tackling infectious diseases. With so many of these things now removed from our lives, it's believed that the immune system becomes unstimulated, almost bored, and starts to look for things to attack—including food particles it would have ignored in the past. Doctors now refer to this theory as the hygiene hypothesis. Whether any of these is truly the reason for food intolerances we'll only discover as research continues, but what we know now is that if you have a food intolerance, identifying it and taking the trigger food out of your diet can help you feel better, look better—and reverse the signs of aging.

THE FOUR FACES OF AGING

Do you have Gluten Face, Dairy Face, Wine Face or Sugar Face?

I think food intolerances are very important, but you don't need to have an official intolerance to a food for it to create changes in your skin. Many foods can do this if you just eat more of the item than your body can tolerate—and the signs are so predictable in the ways that they manifest that over the years I've gotten to a point that I can tell exactly what people have been overeating simply by looking at them.

This is possibly because part of my training as a naturopathic doctor is the study of Traditional Chinese Medicine (TCM), and part of the education in TCM is that the bare face is one of the main ways you can assess and diagnose what is going on within the body. It's often my first clue as to someone's internal wellness. I regularly use TCM face reading as one item in my toolbox to get a clue as to what I suspect might be going wrong for my patients—and then follow up my suspicions using diagnostic tests, which normally confirm the signs I've seen. In fact, it's hard for me to go out without "reading" random people on the street. I want to run up to them and tell them to stop eating dairy or gluten because I can see on their skin that it's doing them harm. There are clear warning signs sent out by the face to alert us to what is going on inside the body—and it's an excellent tool you can use at home to see if you might be overdoing things long before you might feel any other symptoms.

So what would your face tell me about your habits, and how they could be affecting how you are aging? Let's take a look first at the four food-related "faces" I have created from my clinical experience. These are the most common faces I diagnose during my face-mapping sessions. Have a look at the diagrams over the following pages and see if any of them fit the problems you've spotted on your own skin.

Gluten Face

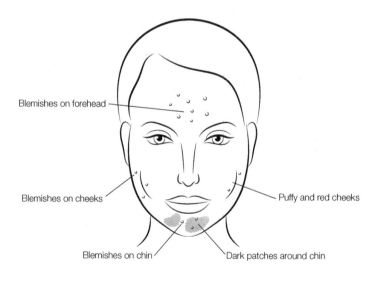

- Blemishes on the forehead
- Puffy cheeks and jowls—your face looks like you've gained weight
- Redness and/or red spots on the cheeks
- Blemishes or darkened patches on the chin

I don't care how many supplements you take, how many peels you have or what you get from a dermatologist to fix your skin; if you have the symptoms of Gluten Face, nothing will make your skin look as good as it can, except removing gluten from your diet.

Gluten is a protein found in foods containing wheat and related grains, such as barley and rye. Oats don't contain gluten themselves but they do contain a similar protein called avenin, which some people can be equally sensitive to. In the scheme of things, gluten is a fairly new addition to our diets (we started eating it about 10,000 years ago, but humans have been around 2.5 million years). This might not have become a problem if we had gradually given our bodies time to get used to it, but between our reliance on carbohydrates at most meals and the fact that gluten makes a very nice thickener and base for flavorings in processed foods, we have very quickly gotten to a point where gluten can be in every meal—if not every mouthful—we consume, and it's likely that our bodies can't cope with such a sudden influx of a relatively new food.

The most important reason to avoid gluten is celiac disease, which we discussed on page 36. If you feel you get symptoms when you eat gluten, it's essential to rule this out as it can lead to some serious health problems if left undiagnosed. Ask your physician to test you. However, testing negative for celiac disease does not mean that gluten is not causing reactions in your system. Research is identifying an emerging group of people who aren't celiac, but who do have a definite reaction to gluten. This was first shown in trials at the University of Maryland,[6] which found that genes and the guts of some people have a definite negative reaction to the presence of gluten (just in a different way from those with confirmed celiac disease) and experts are now calling this problem non-celiac gluten sensitivity. It's estimated to affect six times more people than celiac disease. Clinically I can also tell you that gluten is affecting most, if not all, the patients I see with digest-aging.

Giving up gluten

When you decide to quit gluten, it has to be done well to prevent it from actually causing health problems. The first thing is that you need to know exactly what gluten is in—and the answer is virtually everything. Some of the foods you might not think contain gluten include condiments such as ketchup and soy sauce, soups, ice cream and chips. When you give up gluten, therefore, it's important to read labels very carefully, although when it comes to processed foods you can normally assume if they don't specifically say "gluten free" on the front, it's highly likely to be in there somewhere. I also tell my clients to remember the mnemonic BROWSK—barley, rye, oats, wheat, spelt and Kamut—as these are the types of grains you need to avoid. Remember, though, that there are wheat-based products you might encounter that go by less obvious names—couscous, bulgur wheat (in tabbouleh), freekeh, farro and triticale are all wheat based. If you do choose to eat oats, choose ones that are labeled as "uncontaminated" or state they are gluten free. This means they are not produced in the same area as any gluten products and are not affected by cross-contamination.

If you give up gluten, simply swapping to "free-from" products and eating your normal diet is not the answer. While many wheat-based foods such as bread and cereal are fortified with additional nutrients, gluten-free products don't have to be, and trying to find whole grain versions of gluten-free foods can also be tricky. This can put those eating gluten free at risk of deficiencies, particularly for nutrients such as folate, iron and fiber. The key to quitting gluten and boosting health is to not just swap breads and pastas for processed free-from versions, but instead replace gluten-containing grains in your diet with natural gluten-free alternative grains and seeds that provide healthy doses of fiber and other nutrients. These can include:

- Amaranth
- Buckwheat
- Brown or wild rice

- Chia seeds
- Quinoa
- Teff (an Ethiopian grain)

Choose products such as breads, cereals and flours made from these grains and seeds. Also, use beans and legumes such as lentils or lima beans, and don't forget potato and similar starchy vegetables that can make great side dishes to any meal. Sweet potatoes, for example, are packed with the vitamin A skin needs to thrive, and you can now buy purple potatoes that contain four times the level of antioxidants of white potatoes, making them definitely on the list of skin superfoods. Other members of the tuber family are also good to explore. These are edible plant roots and they include foods such as yams, cassava (also known as tapioca or manioc), and sunchokes (also known as Jerusalem artichokes)—these are particularly good for gut health as they commonly contain the fiber inulin.

Two final suggestions for anyone with Gluten Face. First, I'd suggest taking a supplement of diindolylmethane (DIM). This substance is naturally found in cruciferous vegetables and it helps the body get rid of excess estrogens. High amounts of gluten increase estrogen production, which can be behind some of the fluid retention and breakouts associated with Gluten Face—DIM helps your body rebalance things. Try taking 100–300 mg daily until your symptoms start to disappear.

I also like my Gluten Face patients to use castor oil packs. If you've been eating a lot of gluten you are probably going to be suffering from some level of leaky gut (see page 26). These hot packs that you place across the abdomen help accelerate the healing of that damage. They aren't the tidiest things to use, but here's how make and use one:

1. Get a piece of flannel sheeting and cut it into squares or rectangles a little larger than the size of this book.
2. Apply a layer of castor oil on to the sheet, then apply another layer of sheeting over the top.

3. Wearing clothing you don't mind ruining (castor oil stains clothing) and lying on a thick towel and/or a trash bag to prevent any staining on your bed or couch, apply the pack to the area over your liver (that's on the right-hand side of your front or back, slightly above your waist).

4. Now place a hot-water bottle over the top and lie down for 45–60 minutes.

What's That Rash?

Some people find they develop an itchy, blistery rash on their elbows, shoulders, knees or buttocks after eating gluten. This can actually be a condition called dermatitis herpetiformis, which is a symptom of celiac disease. If you suffer symptoms that sound like this it's important to be tested.

Dairy Face

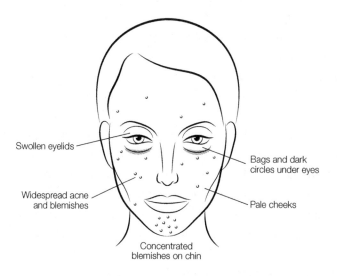

Swollen eyelids

Bags and dark circles under eyes

Widespread acne and blemishes

Pale cheeks

Concentrated blemishes on chin

- Swollen eyelids
- Under-eye bags
- Darkness under the eyes
- Widespread acne and blemishes
- Pale cheeks
- Blemishes around the chin area

Humans are the only species that consume the milk of another animal, and the only species that intentionally drink milk past childhood. It's therefore not surprising that we find it hard to tolerate and that it can have untoward effects in the body.

There are two main substances in dairy that people might react to: sugars and proteins. Lactose intolerance is a reaction to the main sugar in milk, and it is one of the most common food intolerances in the world (particularly in the Asian population). It develops because as we age, we lose the enzymes that allow us to digest lactose effectively. This causes stomach upsets soon after drinking milk. But you can also be intolerant to proteins in milk, and this can be harder to spot, as it's more likely to cause those varied inflammatory symptoms I've talked about than sudden gut distress. You're as likely to suffer fluid retention, fatigue and mood swings as stomach upsets and bloating. If you have Dairy Face, though, there's a good chance that you have issues with milk protein rather than lactose.

Breakouts and red spots on the cheeks can also show that you're consuming too much dairy. Dairy increases phlegm in the body and this affects the lung meridian. In Traditional Chinese Medicine (TCM), signs of this are reflected in the cheek area—some people might also find they lose color in the cheeks or develop a rough texture around the area.

Additionally, dairy causes hormonal changes in the body, particularly rises in insulin and imbalances of estrogen, which show up on the skin in the form of fluid retention. This is responsible for the puffiness and dark circles we see in Dairy Face. Blemishes around the chin are also associated with this hormonal influence, as in TCM the chin is related to the reproductive organs.

One other skin problem often linked to milk is acne. In a study from Harvard University it was found that women who drank more than three servings of milk a day in their teens were 22 percent more likely to develop acne than those who drank less.[7] It's not known exactly why this is the case, but it could be related to hormones in the milk triggering an overgrowth of skin cells that block pores and subsequently trap the bacteria that cause acne.

So, if you do decide to give up dairy, how do you do it well?

Know your dairy

Most of us just think about milk, but it's also yogurt, hard cheese, soft cheese, cottage cheese, crème fraîche, butter, ice cream and Quark. Plus a myriad of processed food items contain dairy products—anything with a creamy taste will have some levels of dairy within it, but surprisingly so can foods such as bread, cereal and processed meats. Protein shakes also commonly include whey or casein.

Find new sources of calcium

So many of my patients ask how to get calcium if they avoid dairy. It's accepted wisdom that we can only get the calcium we need for healthy bones from cow's milk, but that's so very, very wrong. There are over 20 plant-based foods alone that contain calcium. You just need to ensure your diet contains a good variety of alternative sources. Here are some good foods to include:

- **Fish:** Fish with soft bones, such as anchovies and sardines.
- **Vegetables:** Broccoli, bok choy, cabbage, chard, kale, arugula and watercress.
- **Legumes/beans:** Chickpeas, kidney beans, lentils, peanuts and tempeh.
- **Grains:** Amaranth, brown rice, quinoa and teff.
- **Nuts and seeds:** Almonds, Brazil nuts, sesame seeds, sunflower seeds and tahini (sesame seed paste).
- **Fruits:** Figs, rhubarb and calcium-enriched juices.

Find the best alternatives

There are many alternative "milks" on the market that aim to replace cow's milk; some are better than others. The best choices are unsweetened nut and seed milks, such as almond, cashew, coconut or hemp, or, even better, make your own versions (see the recipes on page 260), particularly of coconut milk as it's often found in cans (see page 130 for why this could be an issue). Rice milk can be extremely sugary and so is best avoided, while oat milk can contain very small amounts of gluten.

Some people find that even if they don't handle cow's dairy well, they can tolerate goat's or sheep's milk. These contain slightly different ratios of milk proteins and smaller fat molecules, which the body may find easier to digest.

I usually suggest that people with Dairy Face take evening primrose oil. It's a very powerful anti-inflammatory and can quickly calm any inflammation-based symptoms. You can take up to 500 mg twice a day while your symptoms clear. It can also help to increase your intake of foods rich in vitamins A and E, which help repair the mucous membranes of the gut that can be damaged by dairy. Vitamin A is found in foods such as liver, eggs, carrots and dark green or yellow vegetables and fruits. Vitamin E is found in nuts, seeds and those dark green leafy vegetables again. If you'd prefer to supplement with vitamins A and E, this is best done via a well-formulated antioxidant supplement that balances the levels of each nutrient correctly as antioxidants need to work together. These normally contain vitamins A, C and E. Note: never take more than is recommended of vitamin A supplements—they can be toxic in high does. It's also important not to supplement with or consume excessive amounts of vitamin A if you are, or could be, pregnant.

Wine Face

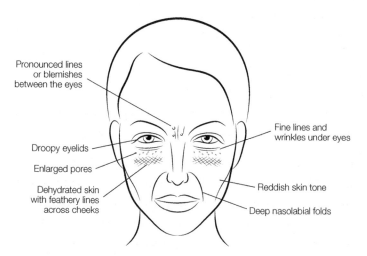

Pronounced lines or blemishes between the eyes

Fine lines and wrinkles under eyes

Droopy eyelids

Enlarged pores

Dehydrated skin with feathery lines across cheeks

Reddish skin tone

Deep nasolabial folds

- Pronounced lines or blemishes between the brows
- Droopy eyelids
- Pronounced fine lines and wrinkles under the eyes
- Dehydrated skin with feathery lines across the cheeks
- Visibly enlarged pores
- A reddish skin tone
- Deep nasolabial folds

I call these symptoms Wine Face, as wine is the most common alcoholic drink consumed by my patients who have this, but it can be triggered by any kind of alcohol. It occurs for many reasons—for starters, alcohol dehydrates the skin, which always worsens the look of fine lines and wrinkles. Alcohol is also high in sugar, which triggers the skin to sag—something you often see first in the thinner skin around the eyes. Darkness under the eyes is a sign in TCM that the kidneys are overloaded, which would be the case when they are struggling to process alcohol. The blemishes or lines between your eyes signify an overload of your liver meridian, which also commonly occurs if you drink more than is good for you.

Making better choices

Reversing the symptoms of Wine Face means, not surprisingly, reassessing your alcohol intake. I advise my clients to give it up completely while balancing the gut afterward, but the good news is if you like to share a drink with friends or unwind with a glass of wine at home, simply making better alcohol choices and consuming it in moderation can be enough to see many of the above aging signs disappear. Try following these rules and see what happens to your skin:

- **Have regular alcohol-free days:** At least four days a week should be alcohol free and you should never drink two days running. Even just one alcoholic drink causes disturbance to the gut lining, and you need to give your body a break from further damage to give that a chance to repair and get over the gut-flammation caused.

- **Choose the purest alcohol you can:** Try to avoid drinks that contain gluten as this creates a double whammy when it comes to attacking the gut lining. Beer is the most obvious of these, but some brands of gin, vodka and whiskey are also made with gluten-containing grains. While some people have no problems consuming these, I think it's better to be safe than sorry and to choose gluten-free spirits such as rum, tequila, or quinoa- or potato-based vodka. For example, you can buy fair trade vodka made from quinoa, which is the first vodka in the world certified fair trade. Wine does not contain gluten but it can be quite sugary so choose drier varieties like Sauvignon Blanc, Pinot Grigio, Merlot or Pinot Noir. The best alcoholic choice you can make is grain-free vodka with soda.

- **Mix alcohol with soda or water, not sugary mixers:** Sugar is also bad for the integrity of the gut lining.

- **Drink water:** Drink at least one glass of water for every glass of alcohol.

- **Choose red wine over white:** Red wine contains more magnesium, more antioxidants, more flavonoids and polyphenols, plus levels of resveratrol that are good for skin.

Research has also found that wines from Sardinia, Italy and Southwestern France have the highest levels of many antioxidants, likely as a result of the grape varieties and traditional production methods used in the regions.[8]

- **Choose organic wines:** Normal grapes are often treated with pesticides, but that won't be the case with organic wines. They are also free from commercial yeasts. Try to choose sulfite-free wines. Many people can react to these preservatives—and if you do have a sensitivity, Wine Face will be even more pronounced. Symptoms such as wheezing, coughing, a runny nose or tightening in your chest after drinking wine are common signs that you are reacting to sulfites, as is a hangover far worse than you think you deserve.

Sugar Face

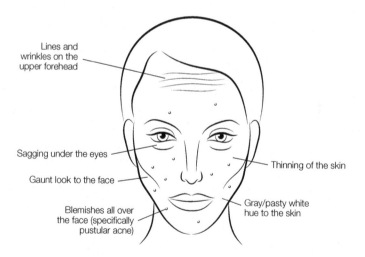

Lines and wrinkles on the upper forehead

Sagging under the eyes

Gaunt look to the face

Blemishes all over the face (specifically pustular acne)

Thinning of the skin

Gray/pasty white hue to the skin

- Lines and wrinkles on the upper forehead
- Sagging under the eyes
- Blemishes all over the face, particularly pustular/cystic acne
- Gaunt look to the face
- Thinning of the skin
- Dark grayish or pasty white hue to the skin

You may know that "a moment of sugar on the lips gives extra inches on your hips," but did you know it can also cause fine lines and wrinkles on your face? Diets full of sugar—and highly refined carbohydrates, which turn quickly to sugar in the system—are a major problem for skin health and contribute to premature aging.

For starters sugar is an inflammatory food, and inflammation is a fundamental cause of aging, but sugar also triggers a process called glycation. When you eat sugar, it is turned into glucose, your body's preferred choice of fuel. However, if you create more glucose than your body needs at any one time and that excess isn't burned or transported into cells to be stored, it remains in the bloodstream, where it can attach itself to collagen, the protein that keeps skin firm and youthful looking. In young skin the collagen fibers are elastic and springy, but if the sugar molecules start to attach to them they harden and become rigid and inflexible. This causes skin to sag and lines and wrinkles to appear.

There's a second issue that occurs with glycation: as the sugars bond to proteins they form compounds called Advanced Glycation End Products (AGEs). It's an appropriate name for them as they make your body older in so many different ways. Not only can these AGEs overwhelm your collagen, leading to sagging, lines and wrinkles, your body also recognizes AGEs are harmful and it mounts an immune defense against them. This triggers even more inflammation, which further attacks the skin.

Sugar also reduces the microcirculation to the skin; it compromises cell turnover and I've even found it affects the fat distribution in the skin. After a while, people who eat a lot of sugar actually get a gaunt look because their face loses the fat that keeps it looking plump. The more sugar you eat, the faster your skin will age—it can make someone in their 20s look 40.

So what do I mean by sugar? Well obviously I mean the sweet white substance that you might sprinkle into tea and coffee, and that makes foods such as cakes and chocolate so appealing to our taste buds. But I also mean refined, white versions of foods such as rice and pasta, which cause sudden rises of blood sugar in the bloodstream, and foods that are high in fructose, which is a type of sugar particularly linked to the production of AGEs. Mostly we associate fructose with fruit, but when it's found in whole fruit it's unlikely to cause much of a problem as it's bound up with fiber, which helps slow its digestion, preventing sudden rushes of sugar into the system. However, a lot of processed foods include highly concentrated doses of fructose in the form of a substance called high fructose corn syrup, glucose syrup, honey or agave nectar. We also can take in concentrated doses of fructose via juices and smoothies. I am a huge fan of juicing, but the main ingredient in any kind of juice should be green vegetables and not fruits—otherwise, you're simply aging your skin with every sip.

Handling sugar cravings

The problem is when you try to give up sugar you tend to want it more and the cravings can be quite overwhelming. To come off sugar successfully, you need to give your diet an overall makeover.

- **Increase your protein intake:** This helps balance blood-sugar levels and prevent crashes that make cravings worse. Every meal needs to have a portion of protein—so meat, fish, eggs or legumes.
- **Don't be afraid of fat:** It helps stabilize blood sugar and keeps you feeling fuller for longer. Healthy sources of fats such as avocados, nuts and oily fish are also anti-inflammatory foods, giving your skin an extra glowing boost while you consume them.
- **Don't give up carbohydrates completely:** Instead switch to whole grains such as amaranth, quinoa, wild rice, teff, millet and buckwheat, which give more sustained blood-sugar levels. This helps to further prevent the blood-sugar peaks and crashes that lead to sugar cravings.
- **Avoid artificial sweeteners:** Not only do they prevent you from losing your craving for sweet tastes, they negatively change the

make-up of gut bacteria. If, once you've rebalanced your sugar levels, you want to sweeten foods, use a natural sweetener such as stevia, xylitol or coconut sugar instead.

- **Consider taking a supplement:** The mineral chromium, the herb fenugreek and the Ayurvedic herb *Gymnema sylvestre* all help to balance blood-sugar levels and may play a role in reducing sugar cravings. You can buy products that combine the three of these in the right quantities.
- **Handle cravings:** If a sugar craving hits, drink a glass of water. It can often help the craving pass.

Got Gas?

While wheat and dairy are the foods most commonly linked to intolerance issues, there's also a subset of people who find that fructose, found in fruit, is their main trigger food. This can be referred to as fructose intolerance but is more accurately named fructose malabsorption. Fructose is normally digested in the small intestine but with fructose malabsorption this doesn't adequately happen— the undigested food ferments in the gut, triggering problems such as bloating, belching or diarrhea. In one trial at the University of Iowa's Carver College of Medicine, 73 percent of people with unexplained abdominal symptoms were found to be actually experiencing this reaction to fructose.[9]

WHAT ELSE IS YOUR FACE TELLING YOU?

It's not just what you're overeating that can impact how old—or young—your face looks. Traditional Chinese Medicine (TCM) also believes that what is happening in the inner body can be determined by examining the face. In TCM, energy flows through the body via a series of channels called meridians. If these are in balance, you remain in good health; if the channels become blocked or imbalanced, health symptoms emerge, and any meridians that are disturbed as a result of diet, lifestyle, stress levels and hormone changes show outward signs on the face. Each part of the face is related to a specific organ system and any disharmony inside of the body will show up on the outside. This could manifest as puffiness, excess lines, color changes, breakouts or zits, itchiness, dull skin or flaky patches in these areas. If you keep getting a blemish or discoloration in the same area over and over again, it's likely that your body is trying to tell you that a part of your system needs attention. Fix that and you might also see an improvement in how your skin looks and behaves.

The illustration below shows exactly what parts of the face correspond to which systems in the body.

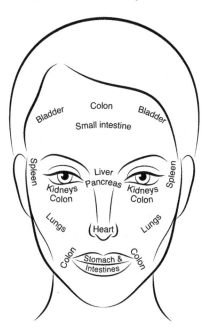

Grab a mirror and spend a few minutes checking your own face. Do any of these areas have lines that don't reflect the level of aging elsewhere on your face—or that you notice seem to come and go? Are there patches of skin that differ in color or texture from the rest of your face or do you always get acne just in one place? Then read on to see what that might be telling you.

The forehead

The forehead is associated with the process of digestion. It is a common area to wrinkle as we age, but if your diet and digestion are poor, the lines on the forehead will be deeper and can even appear on younger skin. The forehead is further divided into three sections. The upper part of the forehead is associated with the bladder meridian, the middle with the stomach and digestion, and the lower forehead with the small intestine.

What might this mean? If the middle or bottom sections of the forehead are irritated, congested, and have blemishes and some lines, this could be related to sluggish digestion as a result of a poor diet. It's also common in those that eat late at night. Trying to eat earlier and carrying out some of the CCP plan in Chapter 1 could see these lines fade—or even disappear.

If your lines or other symptoms are more focused around the top of your forehead, though, I'd be asking about your bladder health. Do you drink enough water? Do you not pass urine often enough— maybe you have a job where you're behind a counter or helping clients all day and just can't get away? Or, are you prone to cystitis? If so, I'd suggest trying a remedy such as cranberry extract, which actually stops the bacteria that cause the infection from attaching to the bladder walls and which may reduce your risk of constant reinfection. If you tackle the root cause of your bladder concerns, you could also find that the forehead lines disappear.

Between the eyes

This area is associated with the liver meridian and is the reason why people with Wine Face (see page 69) see so many of their symptoms manifest in this area. If you're overindulging in alcohol, you may notice vertical lines, acne/blemishes or a reddening develop here. I find it's also common in people who have a dairy intolerance or who consume a lot of processed sugar. I often call this area the "wine and dine" area as it's so closely linked to what we eat and drink. But you can see problems in this area even if people eat what seems like an extremely healthy diet, packed with fruits and vegetables. In this case, the cause is likely to be pesticides and other chemicals that enter the system and overload the liver. I have also seen it in patients who are absorbing too many heavy metals (which can enter the system via water and some of the fish we eat). Try swapping to a more organic diet and following the CCP plan in Chapter 1. Chapter 4's advice about living a less toxic lifestyle may also help reduce the problems in this area.

The brows

I am seeing more and more women with adrenal and thyroid issues caused by hormonal disruptions and stressful lives (I'll talk more fully about these in Chapters 4 and 7), and these commonly show up via changes in the eyebrows. If your eyebrow hair is long and wiry, this could be a sign that you're overly stressed adrenals need support. If you have very fine eyebrow hair or eyebrows that have started thinning throughout, then this is a sign of adrenal exhaustion where those overworked glands have now started to underperform. Left untreated, this can result in subsequent underactive thyroid problems.

Too much sugar can also show up in the brows as it causes insulin imbalances, which overburden the adrenal glands.

The eyes

I have so many patients asking me why they have dark circles under their eyes. Is it genetic, poor sleep, poor circulation, food intolerances, hay fever, iron deficiency anemia? Yes, it can be all of the above, but in TCM, this area relates to the kidneys, and a darkening may indicate that your kidneys are working overtime at eliminating toxins from the body. Obviously alcohol plays a role here but other things that can strain the kidneys are pesticides, dehydration or excessive levels of salt/sodium in the diet. Puffiness around the eyes is a sign that you're holding on to too much fluid—this could be because you're not drinking enough water, or because you're consuming too much salt or sugar (both of which encourage fluid retention). Oh, and check your energy levels—blue circles under the eyes are a common sign of tiredness and exhaustion.

The nose

If you have lots of blackheads, you probably also have poor digestion—and specifically may be affected by low stomach acid levels. If your nose is red or has lots of broken capillaries, this can be caused by drinking too many hot drinks, eating excessive spicy food or consuming too much alcohol. All of these cause the capillaries to dilate, and if this happens too frequently, they can remain enlarged.

The cheeks

In TCM, your cheek area is related to your lungs. If you get redness, irritation or congestion in that area you are also likely to be suffering from sinus issues, asthma or a chronic cough. This area is often also a problem for smokers, but can also be a sign of sensitivity to, or an excess of, dairy, which increases phlegm and therefore affects the lung meridian. If you notice paleness or excessive color in your cheeks or develop a rough texture and/or breakouts in this area, try cutting back on your dairy intake. Pale cheeks can also be linked to low iron levels. If you also suffer low energy, perhaps add some more sources of iron, such as red meat or dark green leafy vegetables, to your diet.

The lips

Do you have constant dry and cracking lips no matter what season it is? It isn't the cold air causing this; it is related to your stomach. If you overload your stomach with irritating foods or processed foods, it will start to break down and lose its normal level of acidity and this will show up on your lips. I'd look carefully for any food intolerances or sensitivities in anyone who regularly suffers from this problem. Cracks at the side of the mouth are a very common sign of low B vitamin levels—this could be because your diet is poor or because your levels of gut bacteria that help make B vitamins are imbalanced. Finally, cracked, flaking lips can also show a deficiency in essential fatty acids, which help maintain healthy cell membranes and associated healthy moisture levels in the body. Increase your intake of nuts, seeds, avocados and oily fish to help counteract this.

The chin

The sides of the chin, along the jawline, are associated with the ovaries and the reproductive organs. Outbreaks around this area are often triggered by hormonal changes and it's the most common place women get blemishes before their period. The middle of the chin, however, reflects bowel health, specifically how well you are eliminating toxins. Congestion here could indicate chronic constipation or incomplete evacuation creating chaos in the gut. Try drinking more water and increasing sources of soluble fiber in your diet to get things moving more efficiently. Some people also find that overdoing gluten can cause slow motility and affect how well your bowels move. Cut back and you might find acne or lines in this area disappear.

Color your face young

Your skin tone can also give away emerging health issues. Whatever your skin color, a healthy youthful skin is uniform in shades and has a glow to it; any deviation from that can be a sign from your body that something is amiss. Here's what to look for:

- **Red areas or a reddish hue:** Most of us associate the color red with the heart and that correlation continues in Chinese medicine, where the color red is associated with the heart and the circulation. Isolated patches of red or an overall red tinge to the face indicates that the blood vessels are widened and in Chinese medicine this is linked to excess—so, you might notice it if you've had a big night out, or a weekend of lots of greasy or spicy foods. In darker skins, you may see a purplish hue rather than redness. Eat clean, swap to a diet of lots of easy-to-digest fresh foods and you'll regain that glow I spoke about.

- **Green or blue:** The saying "green around the gills" for when someone feels a bit ill or nauseous is likely to be true. In Chinese medicine, if your face develops a blue or greenish hue, it's a sign your liver or gallbladder might be struggling. You could be overdoing alcohol, or may be eating too many fatty foods, which can put your gallbladder under strain. However, this shade is also a sign that you might be overloading your body with toxins. Try to reduce your chemical exposure with the tips on how to chemical-proof your life that I include on page 134.

- **Yellow:** This can mean many different things but is commonly linked to problems with the spleen or stomach and is a sign that something is lacking in the body—a yellowish, sallow complexion is often a sign of malabsorption or poor digestion. If I see a patient with a yellowish skin, I also always test them for food intolerance—especially if the yellow is around their eyes or mouth. It really is a telltale sign that something you're eating is not agreeing with you or that your gut health is impaired in some way.

- **Paleness:** Paleness to the skin is often associated with problems in the lung or colon—asthmatics often have much paler faces than my other clients, as do those for whom dairy causes lung congestion. If lung problems get worse or someone develops a more serious condition, such as emphysema, the skin may take on a gray or ashy tone. Paleness is also associated with excessive stress as the blood diverts to the more important organs.

- **Dark areas:** This is a sign of stagnation or blockages in the organs represented by that part of the face—for example, dark circles under the eyes often mean the kidneys or bladder are under pressure; a darker patch of skin around the chin means your bowels need some stimulation.

I hope you've learned in this chapter just how quickly what you eat can show as the signs of aging on your face if it's a food that doesn't agree with you—and how fast things might reverse if you change that. Face reading is an incredible area of medicine and the blueprints I have developed over my years of clinical practice really can allow you to pinpoint changes that can alter how young—or old—your face looks, extremely quickly. In fact, why not photograph your face now so you have something to compare it to once you've tried the plans within this book. Put the before and after pictures next to each other and you'll then be able to clearly see what's changed on your skin. This will also give you a clear indication that things are working beneath the surface to create more lasting changes that aren't usually so readily revealed, such as the changes triggered by the major aging influence we're about to discuss next: inflammation. You might not have heard of it, but it's likely that you're already suffering from it.

CHAPTER 3

INFLAMMATION— THE FIRE WITHIN

Inflammation is the silent epidemic affecting our bodies today. Whether it's caused by what's going on in the gut or something else in your lifestyle, if you have it, you will be aging faster than you should—and the more inflamed you are, the quicker that aging is going to happen. This idea is now so absolute among health professionals, particularly those studying how the body gets older, that many researchers now refer to inflammation as inflamm-aging.

The easiest way to think of inflammation is that it's like a burning fire. Just as a fire in the forest can quickly change from being a slow-burning smolder to a fast-burning inferno destroying everything in its path, that's what can happen in your body with inflammation. The internal fire can eventually get out of hand, affecting every cell in the body and causing us to age faster than we would normally.

I find that outside of the medical profession most people haven't heard of inflammation. If you have heard of it, you may not know exactly what is it and definitely have no idea that it's being linked to not just the facial signs of aging you see in the mirror, but also almost all of the symptoms that plague the body as it gets older, such as aches and pains, middle-age spread and even serious illnesses such as Alzheimer's disease, cancer and heart disease. You also probably have no idea that you have it, but it's been suggested that in Western society, almost everyone over 40 suffers some form of inflammation.

That's certainly true of the patients I see in my clinic—I don't think I've come across anyone who doesn't have some signs of inflammation—which makes it extremely likely that it's affecting you too. In fact, if you do or have any of the following, you'll certainly have some degree of inflammation in your system: smoke, drink alcohol, carry extra weight, live a stressful life, don't sleep as much as you should, suffer any kind of allergy, including hay fever or rhinitis, have skin problems, such as acne, rosacea, eczema, dermatitis or psoriasis, have back pain or joint ache, or have chronic health conditions, including asthma, type 2 diabetes, gum disease or any of the gut problems I discussed in Chapter 1 ... I could go on but I think that's enough for now. I'm guessing I've already just convinced an awful lot of you that you need to read on.

INFLAMMATION EXPLAINED

If you've ever cut or burned yourself, sprained your ankle, or pulled a muscle, you'll have felt inflammation—it's the sudden redness, swelling and heat that occur in an area when it's hurt or damaged and it's your body's attempt to protect itself. In this instance inflammation is a good thing, a sign of just how remarkable your body can be in the face of a threat to its safety. Within seconds the whole body marshals a legion of defenses that all play a role to protect your body from further damage.

To start with, damaged cells in the area produce chemical messengers called cytokines and prostaglandins that send signals to the rest of the body telling it that it's under attack in some way. The messages these chemicals send out start the inflammation reaction. First, they cause tiny blood vessels around the damaged area to dilate, opening up the circulation so blood flow increases and the body can pull everything it needs for healing into the area. The cells become more permeable so that immune cells that attack potential infections can move into the spaces in between them ready to fight. Another set of messenger called leukotrienes then get to work. The job of these is to call the cells of the immune system in to attack any potential infection or danger and send them where they need to go. Fluids carrying those immune cells then flood the area—and the buildup of this causes swelling that cushions and protects the damaged tissue but also stimulates nerve endings that send pain signals to the brain. When the body finally feels it's safe from attack, anti-inflammatory chemicals move into the area. It's a truly incredible system, and without inflammation the body would never heal from injury or infection.

In a perfect world, the only type of inflammation our bodies would encounter would be this positive, emergency response. It would last a few hours or days until the body started to heal and then the anti-inflammatory system would move in and everything would calm back down. But that isn't what's happening; instead our bodies are developing a chronic form of inflammation that triggers a mild form of this reaction day in, day out. When this happens, the impact can be very different from the positive, healing situation described above. In chronic inflammation, reactions that are positive turn negative; the balance of prostaglandins, leukotrienes and cytokines tips so those that cause inflammation become more prevalent and more active—and their anti-inflammatory colleagues that normally mop up the damage simply can't cope. Inflammation gets triggered over and over again—and never gets switched off. The damage this causes manifests all over the body, but I'm specifically going to talk about how it might affect your skin:

- Those dilated blood vessels can lead to redness and the heat they create can trigger rosacea in those prone to it. In time, they can remain open, leading to broken blood vessels on the face that create an aging, uneven skin tone.
- The swelling that cushions tissues can cause puffiness and bloating in the face, leading to under-eye bags and dark circles.
- That opening of the cell walls that lets immune cells get where they need to do their job also makes the cells more vulnerable to free radical damage—a primary cause of aging.
- The prostaglandins, leukotrienes and cytokines released can themselves directly damage the skin. For example, an inflammation-causing cytokine called tumor-necrosis factor alpha (TNF-α)

directly inhibits collagen synthesis and increases levels of a substance called matrix metallopeptidase (MMP-9) in the body, which actively causes collagen destruction. Another inflammatory cytokine called interleukin-1 alpha (IL-1α) actually causes the skin to overproduce pigmentation-producing chemicals that cause age spots and darker patches that age the skin tone. Most of us know that UV rays damage the skin and it's interesting to note that the way they do this is to trigger the release of these exact same inflammatory chemicals. You wouldn't put your skin in the sun every day unprotected (at least I hope you wouldn't), yet when we cause inflammation in our bodies from within we're unknowingly triggering these same damaging reactions to occur every minute of every day.

It's no wonder, therefore, that back in 2008 when a dermatologist called Carl Thornfeldt wrote a paper in the *Journal of Cosmetic Dermatology*,[1] he stated that "chronic inflammation is the common denominator in many mucocutaneous pathophysiologic processes including extrinsic skin aging." In plain English, what he was saying was "inflammation makes your skin age." And in the years since Thornfeldt's paper was published we've learned it's even worse than he feared; it's now known that the link between inflammation and premature aging goes far deeper than the damage done directly to the skin.

The word "inflammation" comes from the Latin *inflammatio*, which means "set alight," and that's a very good way to describe what it does in the body. As I said, it's like a little fire smoldering in the body and the chemicals it releases are like smoke spreading in every direction, getting deep, deep into wherever they can travel—just as smoke gets into everything after a fire. Think of inflammation as a center point—it damages the skin directly but it causes changes in hormones that determine how fast—or slow—we age; it causes changes in digestion that cause all those gut problems associated with faster aging that I discussed before; it changes the gene expression in ways that promote aging—and all of those affect the skin. But we also know that inflammation affects the body deep down inside the cells.

THE TELOMERE CONNECTION

Time for a very quick biology lesson: every cell of your body contains strands of DNA called chromosomes. The cells in your body are constantly regenerating—it's estimated that most cells in your body are less than 10 years old; some, such as the cells lining the wall of the gut, might only be five days old, while the average skin cell lasts just a month because skin cells turn over so often. To regenerate, the cell creates an exact copy of itself, including the chromosomes and the entire DNA contained within it. Every time this happens, though, a tiny cap on the end of the chromosome called a telomere shortens a little. Telomeres are your DNA's protection; imagine them as caps on the end of your shoelaces—if they fell off, the shoelace would unravel and wouldn't perform well, which is exactly what would happen to your chromosomes and DNA. Without telomeres, as the cells copy the chromosomes could unravel, fuse together or start to become damaged, causing flaws and mutations that stop it from functioning correctly or that can even be associated with diseases such as cancer.

The body obviously does not want this and, as such, when the telomeres get to a certain length the cell realizes that it's at a point where these genetic mistakes have, or could, start to creep in and it shuts down the cell to prevent it from potentially making damaged copies. The cell then either dies or goes into a state called senescence, where it's still alive and functioning but can't be replaced. That is the process of aging. However, there's a sting in the tail. Cells in senescence emit higher levels of free radicals and inflammatory chemicals than thriving, replicating cells; the more cells you have in senescence, the faster you age.

Protecting telomeres to try to delay when they reach this "end point" is, therefore, the focus of much anti-aging research. The shorter your telomeres are, the faster the cell gets to the point where it can no longer function well and the faster you age—and vice versa: those with longer telomeres age more slowly. Part of what determines telomere length is believed to be genetic, but it can also be manipulated via the foods you eat, the lifestyle you lead and the damage that your cells are exposed to each day. And guess what? Inflammation attacks the telomeres, causing them to shorten faster than they should. Protecting against inflammation therefore helps protect against aging at a fundamental cellular level.

WHAT CAUSES CHRONIC INFLAMMATION?

Exactly why the inflammatory response goes out of control isn't known, but one theory is that just as the lifestyle we live is wreaking havoc on our gut, we're also living a lifestyle that constantly exposes our immune system to sources of inflammation. This constant drip, drip, drip–style attack floods the system, so the anti-inflammatory response can no longer kick in to stop it from happening.

One source of these inflammatory responses is poor gut health— to remind you, if you have the wrong balance of gut bacteria you produce lower levels of inflammatory chemicals and bacteria thrive that actually release pro-inflammatory ones. Inflammation can also be related to poor nutritional status—if you don't absorb nutrients correctly, you won't have the internal defenses to tackle inflammatory free radical damage correctly. Food intolerances create a clear inflammatory reaction in the body. But, most importantly of all, if you have any damage to the gut lining you will be releasing molecules into the bloodstream that trigger your immune system to mount a full inflammatory attack. When the gut starts to heal, levels of inflammation will naturally start to fall in your system, which is why I suggest everyone carries out the Gut-Balancing CCP Plan (see page 37) before doing anything that you read here.

While it is a major contributor to inflammation, however, poor gut health isn't the only way to increase your inflammatory load. Some of the things we do, and some of the things we eat or drink, also imbalance the ratio of inflammatory chemicals we produce, causing our bodies to produce lower levels of anti-inflammatory chemicals than we need and increasing the levels of pro-inflammatory ones. So, what are these inflammation triggers? Below are eight of the most significant that might be affecting you. Remove these from your life and you lower your risk of inflamm-aging.

1) The Ultimate Agers

By this I again mean gluten, dairy, sugar and alcohol. If you've started the Gut-Balancing CCP Plan (see page 37), you will have already eliminated these from your diet, but to keep you focused here are more reasons why you should. As well as causing damage to the gut, all four of these foods are specifically linked to a greater risk of inflammation. Exactly why varies for each food, but here's a short explanation:

- **Gluten:** If you have a sensitivity to gluten, eating it will clearly trigger an inflammatory reaction in your body, but Danish research[2] has also shown that, in animals generally, eating gluten increased levels of inflammatory cytokines in the system. Even if you don't think gluten upsets your gut, it's likely to increase inflammation and it should be removed from your diet if you're trying to reduce inflamm-aging.

- **Dairy:** In a body with no reaction to dairy, studies show it can have an anti-inflammatory effect.[3] The problem is, many of us do have sensitivities or allergies to dairy so that this benefit is likely to be overridden by our own body's reaction to it. That, combined with its links with acne, an inflammatory condition, and the fact that milk triggers a rapid release of insulin, which can be linked to inflammation, leads me to class cow's milk dairy as an inflammation promoter.

- **Sugar:** When you eat sugar your body releases the hormone insulin—and insulin triggers the release of inflammatory markers. High blood sugar also causes the production of free radicals that damage cells—and remember it's damaged cells that send out the distress signals that trigger the inflammation response. As with the signs of Sugar Face, it's not just the obvious sweet foods that cause problems—refined carbohydrates that the body turns quickly into glucose (aka those with a high GI, or glycemic index) also cause an inflammatory reaction. In fact, researchers at the University of Sydney in Australia found that eating a high GI meal raises levels of inflammatory markers three times higher than a low GI one.[4] And remember those telomeres (see page 86) we're trying to protect? Recent work from the University of California at San Francisco showed that people drinking 8 oz (225 ml) of sugary soda a day had telomeres equivalent to people almost two years older.[5]

- **Alcohol:** Not only does alcohol increase levels of insulin causing the same problems as sugar, it also inhibits an enzyme called delta-6 desaturase. This is the enzyme the body uses to turn plant-based sources of omega-3 fats, such as flaxseed, into inflammation-fighting compounds. In certain circumstances, delta-6, as I'll call it, also has the ability to convert omega-6 fats, which are normally inflammatory, into anti-inflammatory substances. The higher your levels of this essential enzyme, the less inflammatory your body is likely to be. In fact, it's so important that low levels of delta-6 are thought to be one of the key factors in aging. Drink alcohol, however, and your levels of delta-6 will never be optimal.

2) Eating the wrong fats

As you may know, natural fats come in three main types: saturated fats, monounsaturated fats and polyunsaturated fats. When it comes to inflammation, the message regarding two of these is simple: mono-unsaturated fats, found in foods such as olive oil, nuts, seeds and avocados, help reverse inflammation and you should include plenty of these in your diet. Saturated fats, found in dairy products and meats, can increase inflammation so you should limit levels of these in the diet by restricting your intake of dairy products, choosing less fatty cuts of meat and removing any visible fat from the meats you do eat.

Polyunsaturated fats, though, are a little more complex. These can be anti-inflammatory if they contain mostly omega-3 fats (as oily fish and flaxseed do) or pro-inflammatory if they contain high levels of omega-6 fats, as many margarines and vegetable oils such as sunflower oil do.

The reason for this is twofold. First, omega-6 fats are high in a substance called linoleic acid, which, after you eat it, turns into an inflammatory substance called arachidonic acid in your body. This is the substance that your body uses to produce the inflammatory forms of prostaglandins, leukotrienes and cytokines that cause havoc in your system. The more omega-6 fats you consume, the greater your ability to manufacture these inflammation-causing messengers. When you eat omega-3 fats, a similar conversion reaction occurs. But in this case your body converts substances called EPA and DHA (two types of omega-3 fatty acids) into anti-inflammatory forms of prostaglandins, leukotrienes and another group of anti-inflammation-fighting compounds called resolvins and protectins.

The problem is both groups use the same types of enzymes to make the conversion—the two types of fat, therefore, compete for the limited supply of these that we have. Normally omega-6 wins—partly because it's simply more powerful biologically, but also because our diet is flooded with it. Much of the processed food we consume is produced with grain or vegetable oils, which are high in omega-6, and the cattle and farmed fish we eat are often fed grain-based feeds rather than feeds based on grass or algae that they used to consume. The result is our intake of omega-6 far exceeds that of omega-3. In fact, it's now estimated that the average Western diet contains 15–16 times more omega-6 fats than omega-3s—when the correct ratio should be no more than 5:1. Adjusting this ratio is important to fight inflammation. Note, though, I say adjust: omega-6 fats are called essential fats for a reason; we absolutely need them for good health, it's just a case of getting the balance right.

The final type of fat to avoid is trans fats. Formed when oils go through a process that makes them harder, there is now no doubt that trans fats are inflammatory, bad for health and must be avoided in any diet. Thankfully, because the evidence for this is so strong, many manufacturers, particularly in the UK and Europe, have removed trans fats from food, and in June 2015 the US Food and Drug Administration also announced it was giving companies three years to phase out trans fats from foods. Until that full phase-out happens, still be cautious.

You might not realize you are eating trans fats if you go by the label. Labeling law means that if a product contains less than 0.5 g of trans fat a serving, a company can legally label that product as having zero trans fats. But reading the ingredients list tells a different story. In a recent US study, 84 percent of the products labeled zero trans fats had some in their formulation.[6] It's therefore important to read ingredient listings—particularly on cookies, crackers, prepared meals and many processed goods. If you notice the words "hydrogenated" or "partially hydrogenated" fats it means that the item contains trans fats and is best avoided. Also, watch out for interesterified fats. These were brought in to replace trans fats and little is known about them, but some preliminary studies are showing a link with inflammation. Also, therefore, avoid anything with the words "high stearate" or "stearic rich" fat on the label.

3) Excess weight

If you're carrying extra pounds, you're going to have extra inflammation. Fat, particularly fat that collects around the tummy, emits inflammation-causing cytokines. Obese women can have levels of C-reactive protein (CRP) over six times higher than those of a normal weight; men tend to have lower levels, but can find their CRP levels are double that of someone of a healthier weight.[7] Until recently, the reason for this link between weight and inflammation was a mystery, but in 2013 a team of researchers in Texas found something fascinating. They discovered that fat cells act like they are infected with a virus or bacteria and actually produce chemicals that send out distress signals. These lead your immune system to think the cell is under attack, triggering it to start an inflammatory response.[8] Inflammation and weight are also involved in a vicious circle of dependence—the more you weigh, the higher your inflammation, but regardless of weight, the higher your level of inflammation, the harder you'll find it to lose weight. Inflammation stops your body from listening to signals from insulin, which controls blood sugar and interferes with your production of the hunger-suppressing hormone leptin. Start to tackle your weight and you will lower inflammation— start to lower inflammation and you may find it easier to lose weight.

4) Environmental allergies

I have already explained the role that food-related reactions play in the formation of chronic inflammation, but most of us would never dream that our annual bout of hay fever, the itchy skin from playing with a cat or the stuffed-up nose and chest tightness after cleaning and churning up dust could be making us old before our time. If, however, you are allergic or intolerant to something in your environment, your body mounts an inflammatory response to fight it just as it does with a trigger food. Each reaction increases the inflammatory load on your body and your risk of inflamm-aging. Ironically, those who suffer extreme allergic reactions to, say, bee or wasp stings, are less likely to be affected than someone who merely gets a bit of a runny nose when they inhale dust or who suffers with hay fever each summer. People with severe allergies actively seek to avoid their trigger, whereas those with mild allergies either just get on with things or mask the symptoms with an antihistamine. If you suffer allergies—to food or other substances—healing the gut can help reduce the severity of your response and lower your level of inflammation, but finding out what you're reacting to and trying to limit—or even eliminate—your exposure to it is the most effective solution.

5) Stress

The more stress and anxiety you experience, the more inflamed your body is likely to become. In fact, recent trials at Ohio University found that even dwelling on past stressful experiences causes levels of C-reactive protein (CRP—that marker of inflammation) to rise.[9] Why is simple, but goes back to the dawn of time. When our Neanderthal ancestors experienced the stress response they were normally at threat from physical attack and as such their bodies primed the immune system in case it was needed to fight any injury sustained. Now, even though there's no physical danger to the majority of stresses we face, our bodies still mount that same inflammatory response. This isn't a problem if you only suffer the odd bout of stress, but when stress becomes chronic, problems occur. Normally the stress hormone cortisol plays a role in shutting down inflammation, but research from Carnegie Mellon University recently showed that during prolonged stress, it fails. Instead the immune cells actually become resistant to the signals cortisol is sending out and don't switch off the inflammatory response.[10] Frequent or chronic stress therefore helps set up chronic inflammation.

6) Poor sleep

When researchers at Emory University School of Medicine measured levels of inflammatory markers, they found a strong link between how well people slept and the levels of the chemicals in their body—the highest levels were found in those who were sleeping fewer than six hours a night.[11] Sleeping six to nine hours a night was linked to the lowest inflammation risk, although I think everyone should aim for at least seven hours. If you have trouble sleeping, have a look at some of the stress-reducing and sleep-improving tips in Chapter 6—they could help turn things around for you.

7) Smoking

This is one of the primary ways to trigger premature aging in skin. In fact, it's my experience that the average smoker can look up to 10 years older than a non-smoker, and studies have shown that if one twin smokes and the other doesn't, the damage is so obvious that 57 percent of plastic surgeons can spot a smoking twin from a picture of their face.[12] I can do exactly the same thing—smokers have more bags under their eyes, more wrinkles, particularly around their lips, and less firm skin, particularly around the jawline, than non-smokers. Smoking also causes free radical damage and triggers the release of a protein called MMP-1, both of which directly attack collagen and elastin levels—and it also directly triggers inflammation. Every time smoke enters your lungs, it irritates the delicate cells within them; those cells see this irritation as an attack and, as with so many other factors that I've talked about here, that irritation triggers an inflammatory response. If you do smoke, quitting is one of the most important things you can do for your health and looks.

Do You Have Inflammation?

If you do any of the eight things above or have been diagnosed with any condition that ends in the letters "itis"—like gingivitis or dermatitis—which signifies an inflammatory cause, you probably have inflammation. But, it is also possible to test your levels. The most common test used measures levels of C-reactive protein, which is produced by your liver in response to inflammatory signals sent out by your immune system. Personally, though, I wouldn't recommend CRP testing—inflammation is now so prevalent, I would just assume that it is there and simply work on restoring your inflammatory balance using the tips in the plan on page 96.

8) Being sedentary

If you're lying on the sofa reading this book, I'm afraid to say you're contributing to your inflammatory load. A study published in 2012 by a team at the UK's University of Leicester found a clear association with the amount of time women spent sitting and their levels of inflammation.[13] Spanish researchers found a similar trend in men in 2014.[14] Exercise can help counteract some of the inflammatory load caused by sitting (and I'll explain the difference between aging exercise and anti-aging exercise in Chapter 6), but if there's one thing that I predict will become part of anti-aging advice in the future it will be to stand up whenever you can. At work get up and walk around the office for a few minutes at least once an hour; even better, get a standing desk and work for a few hours a day on your feet. In the evening, try to stay active a couple of nights a week rather than just lying on the sofa and watching the latest hit series. I'm not saying stand all day, every day—the aches and pains that might cause can create their own issues with inflammation—just don't spend all your working, and leisure, hours sitting if at all possible.

THE INFLAMMATION-FIGHTING CCP PLAN

If you still need convincing how big a role fighting inflammation can play in reversing inflamm-aging, let me tell you about an experiment conducted back in 2007 by experts at Stanford University.[15] They managed to formulate a skin patch that switched off a compound called NF-kappa-B that fundamentally controls many of the inflammatory processes linked to skin aging. They put the patch on some mice and observed what happened to their skin, and they found it thickened by 75 percent. By switching off inflammation, they managed to stop further age-related decline of the mice's skin and actually reversed the damage that had been done so far. There's a catch with this plan, though—NF-kappa-B is involved with hundreds of genetic reactions in the body—as yet, no one knows what harm switching it off might cause, so forget about putting this book down and just waiting for the magic patch to appear at your local Sephora—it's probably never going to happen. However, there are many natural, health-promoting ways you can fight this silent attacker.

Using this plan

This plan is designed to run alongside the changes you made following the Gut-Balancing CCP Plan (see page 37). If you haven't started that plan yet, it's important to do it for at least four weeks before you begin introducing the steps discussed here. Following the Gut-Balancing CCP Plan will also already have ensured that you have eliminated gluten, dairy, sugar and alcohol—aka the Ultimate Agers—from your diet, which will already have started to reduce your level of inflamm-aging. The information you learned in Chapter 2 may also have identified any food intolerances, which might also be triggering an inflammatory response, and if you've eliminated these, you will have reduced things further. If you haven't done those things you absolutely must act on this before progressing any further. As I said in Chapter 1, aging fundamentally starts in the gut, and if you haven't removed things that damage this and begun to start the process of healing it, you won't get good results from any of the plans that follow.

As you did with the gut plan, follow each of the steps—Clear, Correct and Protect—in turn. Follow Clear for at least two weeks, before adding the steps in Correct for one or two weeks, then integrate the steps in Protect. If you find you aren't getting the results you want then, just as I did with the gut plan, I'll also suggest some ways to "Power Up" your results if you want to use them. You are more likely to need these if you suffer any clear signs of inflammation such as acne, rosacea, allergies, intolerances, or persistent aches and pains.

Clear

The point of this part of the plan is to remove the primary causes of inflammation in your life to try to prevent the inflammatory response being triggered.

1) Cut back on inflammatory fats

That means avoiding trans fats completely, limiting your intake of saturated fat and, most importantly, reducing your intake of foods excessively high in omega-6 fat. As I explained on page 89, the imbalance between levels of omega-3 and omega-6 fats in our diets is believed to be one of the primary causes of inflammation, and rebalancing this level is essential to create an anti-inflammatory, anti-aging state in your body. The absolute best way of doing this is to stop consuming oils and spreads that deliver concentrated sources of omega-6 fats, and avoid the processed foods that contain them. Instead, swap these for oils and spreads with a higher percentage of monounsaturated, omega-3 or other healing fats.

- **Avoid:** Oils made from corn, palm, peanut, safflower, soybean and sunflower; margarines and polyunsaturated spreads.
- **Eat more:** Oils made from avocado, coconut, flaxseed, linseed, macadamia, olive and canola.

2) Heal your body

Hopefully you now understand how many of the minor health problems we put up with day by day can actually be associated with increasing your risk of aging—and potentially even developing more serious conditions later in life. Because of that, I think that anyone suffering from even minor health problems that increase the risk of inflammation should try to find the root cause. Conditions that should be explored include:

- **Aches and pains:** If you have pain, you have inflammation. If you're suffering from regular back pain, joint pain, sports injuries, etc., then instead of just masking the symptoms, try to find out what might be behind them by seeing an acupuncturist or naturopathic doctor for acupuncture, or a physiotherapist, osteopath or chiropractor. If your pain is more arthritic, you might actually find that lowering inflammation sees an end to many of your symptoms.
- **Allergies:** Anyone who regularly suffers irritating symptoms such as sneezing, wheezing, cough, stuffed-up nose, itchy or swollen eyes, post-nasal drip, skin rashes, dermatitis, isolated patches of dry skin or eczema probably has some kind of allergy

or other reaction to something in their diet or surroundings. I've already spoken about food allergies and intolerances at length in Chapter 2, but, don't forget, there are a lot of common non–food related allergens out there. Airborne particles of pollen, dust, mold or pet dander (while many of us think we are allergic to the fur of animals, it's actually skin cells attached to the fur that most react to) often cause nasal symptoms such as sneezing, wheezing, runny nose, stuffy nose or cough, while skin reactions such as eczema, dermatitis or hives may be more associated with perfumes, colorants and chemicals from the fabrics, washing detergents, toiletries, etc., that our skin comes into contact with every day. Often these reactions occur quite quickly after exposure to the allergen and so you can normally determine for yourself what the problem is by keeping a food diary (see page 56). If you aren't sure, suspect you may have multiple allergens or want confirmation of your food diary suspicions, you can have a skin prick test. Normally done via the inside of your arm, you have a tiny amount of the suspect substance(s) applied to your skin. The skin is then pricked to introduce this into the body. Your body will launch an inflammatory response to the invader, which shows as reddening and a welt or lump forming in the area. If you don't react, it's likely you aren't allergic to the substance; if you do, it's important to avoid it from then on to stop your symptoms and lower your risk of inflamm-aging.

- **Anything that ends in "itis":** "Itis" is medical shorthand for a condition that involves some level of inflammation, so conditions such as gingivitis (gum disease), arthritis (joint inflammation), dermatitis (itching and inflammation of the skin), gastritis (inflammation of the stomach lining) all involve some level of inflammation and will therefore be adding to your inflammatory load. Ask your dentist, doctor, dermatologist or another medical professional if there is anything you can do to actually cure your condition—or at least stop it from triggering—rather than just taking medication to reduce the symptoms.

- **Poor sleep:** As studies show, just one night of poor sleep increases your levels of inflammatory markers and raises the inflammatory load on your body. If you sleep poorly regularly, it's very important for your health to change this—you'll find some specific sleep-boosting tips in Chapter 6.

3) Check your weight

Carrying fat will raise inflammation and losing any extra pounds will reduce it. In fact, in a trial at the Fred Hutchinson Cancer Research Center in Seattle, losing just 5 percent of body weight triggered huge drops in levels of inflammatory markers by as much as a third (and even more when subjects combined diet with exercise to lose the pounds).[16] The more weight the women lost, the more their level of inflammation fell. So do you need to lose weight? It's possible—at the time of writing, the World Health Organization says that 39 percent of the world's population are overweight and 13 percent are obese. According to the Centers for Disease Control and Prevention (CDC), more than a third of US adults over 20 years are obese; if you include overweight adults, that figure balloons to 69 percent of Americans. In the UK alone, one in four people is obese[17]—yet only 6 percent of the population think this might be the case.[18] The fact is that many of us have lost sight of what a healthy weight looks or feels like and so don't realize that we are actually carrying additional inflammatory pounds. That's why I suggest checking the following two measures:

- **Your waist measurement:** A waist that measures over 35 in (88 cm) in women or 40 in (102 cm) in men is associated with greater inflammation—and a greater risk of health problems overall. If your waist measures more than this, you will have inflammation. Before you wrap the tape measure around the skinny part where your skirt or pants button up, note that medically the waist is considered to be the point around or just under your navel. You should measure here first thing in the morning so it's not affected by any bloating you might experience later in the day. Breathe out and relax your stomach to get a true measurement.

- **Your BMI:** It's not a perfect measure if you are an athlete or naturally carry a high muscle mass, but for the general population, Body Mass Index (BMI) does give a good basic idea of whether your weight is healthy or not, especially in conjunction with waist measurement. To find your BMI, divide your weight in kilograms by your height in meters squared. Now, check your result against the below:
  - » 18.4 or under—you are underweight
  - » 18.5–24.9—you are a healthy weight
  - » 25–29.9—you are overweight
  - » 30 or over—you are obese

If you score highly on both of those measures, then losing weight will help reduce your level of inflamm-aging. But this doesn't mean I want you to go on any kind of crash or fad diet to do it—that can be stressful to the body and trigger health issues of its own. Being very underweight is also linked to higher inflammation. Instead, aim to balance your weight by eating real, unprocessed foods, and focusing your meals on protein, vegetables and whole grains. If you want to lose weight, cut out any foods to which you're sensitive as these may stall your efforts. And listen to your appetite: eat when you are hungry, stop when you are full. For help in doing this, follow the Age-Reversing Eating Plan that starts on page 204. Also, start moving—exercise is a great way to naturally balance your weight. Even if you don't need to lose weight, I would still strongly suggest you exercise—moving your body lowers levels of inflammation of its own accord but also helps fight it in secondary ways, such as improving sleep. Exercise can help protect the body against many illnesses that trigger inflammation; it even makes you less sensitive to allergens.

Correct

Once you've started to remove sources of inflammation in your diet, you can start adding in things that have anti-inflammatory effects.

1) Up your intake of healthy fats

While trans fats, saturated fat and omega-6 fats cause inflammation, other fats counteract it. Specifically monounsaturated fats such as those in nuts, seeds, avocados, olives and the oils made from these, and the omega-3 fats found in foods such as oily fish, flaxseed and walnuts. Studies have shown that when you consume omega-3 your body's response to inflammation subtly changes. For starters it can use the fatty acids EPA and DHA in these fats to build anti-inflammatory forms of prostaglandins, leukotrienes and cytokines, plus it also produces another set of molecules that actively fight inflammation. Called pro-resolution molecules, these switch off the inflammation process and help the body repair the damage it has done. Two of them, resolvins and protectins, are produced directly from omega-3 oils; the third, lipoxins, are made by your body from omega-6 fats—that's right, in the right circumstances, harmful fats can actually produce a helpful substance. However, this can only happen if levels of EPA and DHA in the body are high. So, how can you add healthy fats? Here are some good sources:

- **Oily fish:** These are the absolute best source of omega-3 fats as they naturally contain high levels of both EPA and DHA. Good sources are salmon, herring, sardines, anchovies, mackerel, fresh tuna, trout, roe and caviar. Note: Farmed salmon is generally quite low in omega-3 fats and is higher in omega-6 fats. Buy wild salmon if possible.
- **Grass-fed meats:** Cows and sheep that eat grass rather than grain-based feed naturally produce meat with higher levels of omega-3 fats.
- **Omega-3 enriched eggs:** Some chickens eat enriched feed that creates eggs with higher than average levels of omega-3 fats.

- **Nuts and seeds:** Walnuts, cashews, pecans, almonds, brazil nuts and pine nuts, along with chia, pumpkin and flax seeds, are good choices.
- **Oils:** Flaxseed oil, canola oil and walnut oil are high in omega-3s.

POWER UP

Take a fish oil supplement. This provides a concentrated dose of omega-3 to the body, and in studies at Ohio State University, people taking a daily dose of fish oil saw their level of inflammatory markers fall by 14 percent.[19] But fish oil also helps counteract inflammation in another way: by reducing your reaction to stress. In the Ohio trial, the anxiety students felt during exams fell by 20 percent while they were taking supplements. Australian studies also showed a decreased stress response when people were taking fish oils.[20] If you believe your stress level is a major contributor to your levels of inflamm-aging, then taking fish oil is an extremely simple step to take to tackle the damage. I'll explore others ways to fight stress in Chapter 6.

Good fish oils clearly state how much of EPA and DHA they contain on the packet—you should be aiming for a dose of 650 mg of the two combined. Purity should also be a concern—large fish from which some companies extract their oils can be contaminated with heavy metals, which then enter your system when you consume the oils. To find a purer oil, look for companies extracting oils from smaller fish, such as anchovies or sardines, which are less affected by heavy metals and/or who clearly state they clean the oil under low temperatures. The gold standard of purity, though, the International Fish Oil Standards Program (IFOS) certification—this means the fish oils are independently tested to ensure they're as pure as possible.

If you're vegetarian, you obviously won't want to t fish oil. However, vegetarian sources of omega-3, ! as flaxseed, canola oil and nuts, aren't as potent. The omega-3 fat they contain, alpha-linolenic acid (ALA), needs converting to EPA to have the optimum anti-inflammatory effect in your body. This process can be hindered if your body is low in the enzymes it needs to carry out conversion. In fact, it's estimated that only 8–10 percent of the ALA in flaxseed actually converts to EPA (and no DHA is produced). A newer supplement called echium oil, made from the *Echium plantagineum* plant, takes fewer steps to convert to APA, which means you are more likely to achieve higher EPA levels when taking it.

2) Know your ABCs

There are a number of superhero vitamins and minerals that especially fight inflamm-aging, and your diet should be high in these.

- **Vitamin A:** This helps my patients who have gut-flammation in the intestines, the lungs and the skin. Those with inflammatory bowel disease, acne and chronic asthma, and lung issues all improve if I spruce up their vitamin A levels for a short time. Good dietary sources include liver, but as you can consume too much of pure vitamin A, it's better to get it from green, orange or yellow vegetables as these convert the betacarotene they contain to vitamin A. It's particularly important not to supplement or consume too much pure vitamin A if you are pregnant or trying to conceive, and no one should exceed more than 1.5 mg daily via food, supplements or a combination of the two.

- **B vitamins:** I always give my patients B vitamins to help them with the "itis" conditions and to help fight gut-flammation generally. The B vitamins also help counteract an extremely inflammatory substance called homocysteine that can build up in the body. Particularly important are B6, B9 and B12. Whole grains are excellent sources of the B vitamins, except B12, which is found in meat and eggs, so vegans need to supplement with this. You need 1.5 mcg a day.

- **Vitamin C:** This significantly lowers levels of C-reactive protein in the body. It's also an effective antioxidant and has anti-inflammatory benefits. It's particularly effective when combined with vitamin E. Good sources of vitamin C include bell peppers, blueberries and kiwi fruit. Vitamin E can be found in nuts, seeds and avocados.

- **Vitamin D:** Low levels of vitamin D have been linked to various inflammatory conditions. It's an important anti-inflammatory as it actually reduces the production of pro-inflammatory cytokines. We mostly make vitamin D from sunlight; it's very hard to get it exclusively in the diet and so I do suggest supplementing with it. The basic recommended dose is 10 mcg (400 IU) daily, but I recommend 50 mcg (2,000 IU) a day if levels are less than optimal (which means a blood measurement of between 85–125 nmol/L), especially in winter or for those who cover their bodies. Vitamin D levels can be checked with a blood test and I recommend you have this done annually to ensure you're getting an adequate intake. Your doctor may test vitamin D levels if you have symptoms of deficiency; if not, you'll have to pay for it to be done privately. You can buy tests that you do at home (www.vitamindcouncil.org/testkit).

3) Use more spices

Many spices have anti-inflammatory effects in the body—ginger, garlic, cayenne pepper, black pepper and chili powder, for example, can all help fight inflamm-aging and you should start adding these liberally to your foods.

However, absolutely *the* most potent spice you can add to your diet is turmeric. My family has been using this spice since I was born for flavoring and it goes in so many dishes—I use it in everything from scrambled eggs to stews and curries; you'll find plenty of examples in the Age-Reversing Eating Plan on page 204. The substance that gives this spice its bright orange color is called curcumin and it acts against inflammation in a multitude of ways. It's been shown to switch off the enzymes needed to produce pro-inflammatory substances, it scavenges free radicals that make inflammation worse and, perhaps most importantly, it acts upon the NF-kappa-B that controls much of the inflammatory cascade.[21] It's so powerful that trials have found curcumin reduces a huge variety of inflammatory markers—and that its action on inflammatory conditions such as rheumatoid arthritis is comparable to painkillers in reducing symptoms[22]—but, unlike painkillers, curcumin also helps fight the root cause of that pain.

4) Eat your antioxidants

As I explained, the cellular damage triggered by free radicals can also trigger an inflammatory response within the body. Antioxidants found in healthy grains and brightly colored fruits and vegetables neutralize free radicals and prevent them from causing damage. It's probably no surprise to hear that people with lower levels of antioxidant nutrients, such as vitamin C and vitamin E, have a greater risk of inflammation than those with healthy levels. The more colorful, varied and antioxidant packed your diet is, the more powerful it is at fighting free radicals and inflammation. I'd therefore suggest eating a wide variety of non-gluten-based grains, different colored fruits and vegetables, oily fish and healthy oils—it's no coincidence that people in some of the longest-living places, such as Japan, Greece and parts of Italy, all follow this kind of plan.

Protect

Once you've cleaned out the bad and added in the good, it's time to ramp up your protection with foods, supplements or lifestyle tricks that actively protect your body against further inflammatory attacks.

Maximize your enzyme boosters

If you want to create a body that's anti-inflammatory most of the time, you need to look after your delta-6 desaturase enzyme. Remember, this is the enzyme that helps you use vegetable sources of omega-3 fats to build the helpful anti-inflammatory forms of prostaglandins, leukotrienes and cytokines—but it also has another essential role. If you have low levels of omega-6, high levels of omega-3s and a healthy supply of delta-6, you can actually turn any omega-6 fats you do eat into anti-inflammatory lipoxins. A balanced diet that supplies healthy levels of vitamin B6, magnesium and zinc all help delta-6 do its job. This is why, even though I exclude gluten from the diet, I don't exclude grains per se; they, alongside dark green leafy vegetables, are good sources of the nutrients you need to fight inflammation.

POWER UP

Think about taking a "bad enzyme" blocker: while delta-6 is a helpful enzyme, it has a couple of evil twins— cyclooxygenase-2 (COX-2) and 5-lipoxygenase (5-LOX). These enzymes are the ones used to produce pro-inflammatory compounds. But some supplements actually block the production of them:

- **Gamma-linoleic acid (GLA):** This is found in supplements such as evening primrose oil (EPO) and borage oil, and in the right quantities it acts to block COX-2 and 5-LOX. It also acts directly on the genetic causes of inflammation, preventing the switching on of genes that produce cytokines—the inflammatory messengers that set the inflammatory cascade in motion. When I give this to patients with dry, irritated skin and eczema it helps them immensely. I recommend a dose of 500 mg twice a day of evening primrose oil until your symptoms start to subside. Do not take more thinking it will boost the beneficial effect—doses of over 3,000 mg a day of EPO will tip the balance between its anti- and pro-inflammatory actions, and may actually trigger inflammation. Also don't take GLA if you are on blood-thinning medications, such as warfarin, or while on some forms of immuno-suppressive medication without the advice of your doctor.

- **Boswellia:** This is one of my favorite supplements to use in patients who come to me with inflammatory issues. It is an Ayurvedic herbal remedy made from tree resin that blocks 5-LOX activity. As an added bonus, it also acts on other pro-inflammatory chemicals including TNF-α (see page 84), which is directly involved with the destruction of collagen. The recommended dose is 300 mg up to three times daily until your symptoms disappear.

- **Pycnogenol:** This extract from the bark of French pine trees is the third remedy I might prescribe to my patients. Again, it is known to block both COX-2 and 5-LOX enzymes. Pycnogenol is also a powerful antioxidant and so helps fight the free radical pathway of inflammation and helps specifically fight against skin aging. In trials it has been found that pycnogenol increases hyaluronic acid synthesis-boosting hydration,[23] and prevents damage to the elastin fibers that help keep skin firm.[24] The recommended dose is 1 mg per kilogram that you weigh—so, if you weigh 60 kg (132 lb), you should take 60 mg.

So that's it; a crash course in the epidemic of aging that is inflammation. I find it quite scary how prevalent it's become in the patients I see and in society generally, but the good news is that once you understand how to reverse it and take those simple steps, your body will respond very well. Just as if you cut out a food to which you're intolerant, you could be amazed at what happens when you start to fight inflammation; problems such as acne and rosacea can reduce, skin tone will improve, and problems such as aches and pains and stubborn weight gain that you thought were part and parcel of the aging process can all start to reverse.

Chances are by now you're very surprised by how much you can change about your body as you age. If so, I'm about to blow your mind: you know those hormonal symptoms you think you have to live with every month, or that you assume are an inevitable part of getting older? They too can be controlled if you just know how—which is what I'm going to discuss in the next chapter.

CHAPTER 4

REJUVENATE YOUR HORMONES

If you suspect you're aging prematurely, it won't just be what you see in the mirror that's affected by that—but how you feel as well. Many of the patients I see come to me because they simply start to look and feel like "crap" as they start to get older—sorry, but that's the word they use to describe what's going on! They've already tried everything else to help reverse this—they've visited their doctor, had endless beauty treatments, but nothing is working. I often say to patients, you spend the first half of your life chasing wealth and the second half chasing health—and when it comes to the problems I'm talking about in this chapter that statement has never been truer. For some female patients the decline starts only at age 50 when menopause begins, for others it begins in their 40s when they enter the state of hormonal flux that is peri-menopause. For some women, though, changes can begin as early as their mid-30s if conditions are right (or rather, wrong!).

It's not just women who get affected by hormonal changes—men also experience fluctuations that affect how they look and feel. Testosterone levels fall and this has a major impact on blood sugar, insulin sensitivity and the function of the adrenal glands, which control much of our hormonal health.

Don't think you're off the hook if you're in your 20s and currently feel completely hormonally healthy—what you do now to influence your hormones will start to show up in your 30s or 40s. As such, it's never too early (or late) to try to balance them.

At whatever age these changes occur, the symptoms are the same. Many female patients tells me they started to feel flat and exhausted, particularly after having children or between the ages of 40–60 when the hormonal decline associated with menopause kicks in. They develop problems sleeping, moods start to change—one minute calm and collected under the face of pressure, the next every little thing seems to be getting them down—and that ability to juggle and keep all the balls in the air vanishes. On top of this come changes to their looks: dull, dry skin that just seems immune to any kind of cream applied to it; a sudden rush of wrinkles; pigmentation changes; and hair and nails that look as sub-par as their "owner" feels. The culprit in all of this is hormones—and the fluctuations in their levels that occur naturally as we get older.

However, there's a difference between natural hormone decline and what's happening to many of us today. What's happening now is that our natural hormonal changes are being worsened by factors in our diet, lifestyle and/or environment. Many of my patients live with this, thinking they need to accept looking and feeling subpar "as natural: I'm getting older," not realizing that actually what they are experiencing is worse than it should be. Some might even seek medical advice from their doctor and be told, "It's natural, there's nothing wrong with you." Again, they feel there's nothing they can do—but that's not the case at all. I can absolutely tell you that those who do something to support the hormonal transition that comes with aging, and/or that take steps to prevent any excessive hormonal imbalances triggered by lifestyle factors, will not only suffer fewer hormonally linked symptoms but a less accelerated rate of aging too.

PIGMENTATION—WHEN HORMONES ATTACK

Before I talk more about hormones themselves, I want to focus a little bit on pigmentation. I've talked about this throughout the book, explaining how sun exposure and inflammation can be linked to an increase in pigmentation (both cause the cells that produce the dark pigment melanin to behave erratically), but when it comes to its development, especially at younger ages, hormones can also be closely involved.

First, the reproductive hormones estrogen and progesterone can trigger it. This is called melasma and it appears as brown or light gray patches of pigmentation that most commonly appear on the face, specifically the forehead, cheeks, upper lip and chin. It usually appears between the ages of 20–50 and is very commonly triggered during pregnancy or in women who are taking the contraceptive pill. Exactly how the hormones trigger melasma isn't yet known, but it is related to the combination of hormonal surges and exposure to sunlight. It's therefore even more important for women using hormonal contraceptives or who are pregnant to use sunscreen.

Stress also causes pigmentation. In this case the issue is caused by an enzyme called tyrosinase. Tyrosinase is used to produce melanin, but it also helps your body produce higher levels of stress hormones. The problem is that tyrosinase does this by oxidation—a process that creates darkening (think of what happens to an apple once it's exposed to the air). If tyrosinase levels are raised in the body, as they will be during stress, not only are they producing more melanin, that melanin is also more likely to darken—and hyperpigmentation can be the result.

Insulin also plays a role in a certain type of pigmentation. If levels of this are high, you can develop patches of dark, thickened, velvety skin on your neck, armpits or groin. This is called acanthosis nigricans and it's a common sign of insulin resistance or even type 2 diabetes. If you have this, it's very important to have your blood glucose levels checked.

It's often said that darker skins don't show signs of aging as early as Caucasian skins do—that's not strictly true. The higher levels of protective melanin in darker skins might mean they don't suffer lines and wrinkles as early as lighter skins do, but they are more prone to pigmentation. In my darker-skinned patients it's often the first sign of aging and one that concerns them greatly.

Balancing hormone levels will help reduce the risk of pigmentation occurring and can often reverse melasma, but if it's already developed there are a number of skincare ingredients that help lighten the pigment. I use products that contain alpha-arbutin (a natural lightener derived from bearberry extract), vitamin C in the form of L-ascorbic acid, kojic acid and licorice extract or burdock root extract, all of which help to inhibit the production of tyrosinase. In Chapter 5 you'll also find some home masks that help keep the skin bright and even-toned.

DON'T SHOOT THE MESSENGER

Hormones are our body's messengers: they give orders. They're like the boss at work telling the cells, their employees, what to do. They're produced by the endocrine glands, which include the ovaries in women, the testes in men and, in both genders, the pituitary, the pineal, the thyroid, the thymus, the pancreas and the adrenal glands—and also by tissues such as fat or the gut lining. To work, they travel in the bloodstream until they reach a cell that listens to their commands. At this point they dock in a hole called a receptor and from there they can tell the cell what to do. While the cell uses the hormone, that hormone breaks down, and once that breakdown is complete the function stops. It takes very little of a hormone to do its job—and this is one reason why imbalances or fluctuations in their levels affect the body so significantly.

When we say the word "hormone," most of us think of the sexual and reproductive hormones—estrogen, progesterone and testosterone. They are the ones we often spend so much of our life feeling the obvious symptoms of, due to problems such as PMS, period pain, acne or effects on libido. But there are hundreds of different hormones in the body, each with an individual role, and even now scientists are still finding new ones. There are hormones that determine your reactions to stress, that help you sleep, that give you energy, that control appetite, that build muscle and that regulate

REJUVENATE YOUR HORMONES • 113

pain. They are involved in absolutely every process within your body, including the aging of the skin. One fun fact: we didn't even have the word "hormone" until 1905 when a doctor called Ernest Starling came up with it—that's how comparatively new our understanding is of all this.

From my clinical experience, the more out of balance your hormones are, the quicker you will age. This might be because the levels of hormones that promote youthful activity in the body have actually fallen or because something is preventing them from working the way they should; or it could be because hormones that age us are being produced in excess in the body and you need to turn down their activity to also turn back time. These issues cause age-related changes all over the body, but I specifically describe the hormonal effect on the skin as being grape-like. When the hormones are at their highest and performing well, you look like a grape—everything is plump (and when it comes to skin, plump is good!). However, as the hormone levels fall, everything sort of deflates and you become more like a raisin. My plan is to keep you grape-like for as long as possible!

Before I explain how to do that, though, I'll explore the hormones in turn—no, not all 100-plus of them, just the ones that are most important when it comes to aging, and specifically aging of the skin. I'll explain exactly what they do, which are the good, the bad—and the dirty hormones—and how you can tell if yours are out of balance.

THE YOUTH BOOSTERS

These are the hormones that make us look and feel younger.

Estrogen

Produced by the ovaries prior to menopause, and then in a weaker form by the adrenal glands and fat cells afterward, estrogen is possibly the most important hormone when it comes to keeping skin feeling and looking youthful. The more estrogen you have in your system, the more collagen you produce and the thicker, and less likely to wrinkle, your skin will be. Estrogen helps skin retain moisture more effectively and stimulates the production of fresh skin cells to replace the dead cells that can build up on skin, making it look and feel dry or dull.

Falling estrogen is one of the prime triggers for noticeable aging in the skin. In fact, the skin thickness declines by 1.13 percent each year after menopause when estrogen levels fall—collagen also decreases by as much as 30 percent in the first five years after menopause, according to one trial.[1] Conversely, however, in research by the University of California at San Francisco, it was shown that postmenopausal women supplementing with estrogen, as many do via hormone replacement therapy (HRT), were less likely to develop drier skin and had fewer lines and wrinkles.[2] (HRT is not recommended for all women; check with your doctor before starting on any estrogen supplement.) However, reaching menopause is not the only reason you might be suffering from falling estrogen levels and aging faster than you should.

Day after day your body is being exposed to estrogen-like chemicals via your diet or environment. Called xenoestrogens, these are part of groups of chemicals known as endocrine disruptors but that I call "dirty hormones." These are chemicals that can disrupt our entire hormonal system. Remember that receptor in the cells that allows hormones to enter and instructs the cell on how to behave? Well, "dirty hormones" trick this receptor into believing they are the real hormone and therefore the cells let them in and they can then act on the cells; they are imitators, liars, something pretending to be something it's not. When this happens your body thinks it's responding to the real thing but it doesn't have the positive, youth-boosting effects on the skin—the effect is not healthy, it's not anti-aging and it's not beautiful. Dirty hormones interfere with hormone levels in all sorts of ways—they can increase levels of unhealthy hormones (such as cortisol), and they can decrease levels of others (such as testosterone or thyroid hormones). They can tell healthy cells to do things they are not supposed to do (such as self-destruct) and they can alter in structure to become substances that are directly harmful to our system. Or simply, they can block the receptor, stopping your real version of the hormone from doing its job. Having dirty hormones in your body can wreak havoc on your entire hormonal inflammatory system.

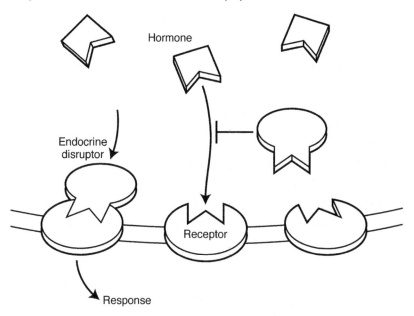

Estrogen is also produced by fat cells—if you're carrying excess weight, this can also increase levels in the body. This might sound like a good thing, considering how good estrogen is for skin, but too much estrogen can lead to a problem called estrogen dominance, which stops our second reproductive hormone, progesterone, from doing all its tasks within the body effectively—and progesterone is also associated with good skin health as it's involved with skin elasticity. Too much estrogen will also interfere with the work of androgens—male hormones, such as testosterone. Women do have low levels of these and they are responsible, among other things, for ensuring the skin produces healthy levels of oils. Testosterone also controls libido—and it's been found that women who have a healthy sex life look up to 10 years younger than those who aren't as sexually active.[3] If your testosterone levels are low, you might miss out on that boost. Finally, remember, those fat cells also pump out anti-inflammatory chemicals that damage the skin. Gaining weight is not a fountain of youth.

In a nutshell, to age well, you need to try to ensure your skin cells are receiving signals from the estrogen that you do produce—and that you have the right levels in your bloodstream. The problem is, that doesn't always happen. Signs that estrogen is imbalanced are:

- **Mental symptoms:** Anxiety, depression-like symptoms, forgetfulness, increased susceptibility to stress and mood swings.
- **Physical symptoms:** Breast tenderness, endometriosis, fatigue, fibrocystic or lumpy breasts, fluid retention—particularly around the wrists and abdomen, hot flashes, loss of libido, night or day sweats, uterine fibroids, vaginal dryness, weight gain around the hips, thighs and arms.
- **Skin symptoms:** Dry skin, faster formation of lines and wrinkles, pigmentation problem, sagging skin.

If you suspect your estrogen levels are imbalanced, and you are in your late 40s to early 50s, your first stop should be your primary doctor who will measure your levels of a hormone called follicle-stimulating hormone (FSH), which rises as menopause nears. If this is high, you are therefore nearing menopause and this is likely to be the main reason behind your problems—although, as I said before, that doesn't mean you can't do anything about it. Following the tips in the CCP plan that follows will still optimize the hormones that you have, helping them act younger and healthier even as menopause approaches. If your FSH is normal, then you aren't officially going into menopause, but that doesn't mean your estrogen levels are not imbalanced for other reasons. In this case, a naturopathic doctor or integrated practitioner would also measure levels of salivary hormones throughout the month, which measures a slightly different form of the hormones than is found in the bloodstream and can pick up problems that one blood test can't. Some practitioners might also add urine testing, which can show if the imbalance is caused by the liver being under strain from exposure to stressors such as environmental chemicals. However, don't worry if you can't access these tests—

following this plan will still help keep the hormones you have healthy and prevent their levels from rapidly going downhill (and your skin following closely behind).

Specifically, exercise helps balance estrogen levels, as does adding natural hormone mimics called isoflavones (found in foods such as soy, peanuts and alfalfa) to your diet. Increasing natural estrogen detoxifiers (via supplements or by including more fiber and cruciferous vegetables in the diet) also helps reduce the effect of xenoestrogens.

DHEA—dehydroepiandrosterone

This hormone is produced by your adrenal glands. I describe it as the "mother hormone to all hormones," meaning your body converts it into other hormones including estrogen and testosterone. That doesn't make it unimportant in its own right, though. Generally DHEA helps maintain bone and muscle strength and is also involved in cognitive function—in terms of the skin, its main role is to control oil production and balance sebum production, keeping the skin hydrated. It also helps increase collagen production; in fact, in one trial when the skin was exposed to DHEA, an amazing 61 different genes controlling collagen function all switched on.[4] Genes that control the production of new healthy skin cells also fired up, possibly explaining why DHEA also helps protect the integrity of the skin's barrier. Levels of DHEA peak at age 35, at which point you're producing 6–8 mg a day; by the time you're aged 70–80, you'll be making 10–20 percent of that. But aging isn't the only thing that can lower DHEA production, and the most common trigger for falling levels is as likely to affect you at age 27 as at age 77, and that's stress. All stress will slightly lower DHEA production, but the most damaging form is chronic, long-term stress that leads to a condition called adrenal fatigue.

The adrenal glands are tiny glands that sit on top of your kidneys. They play a vital role in your overall hormone production and are involved with balancing many of the hormones we're discussing in this section. Poor adrenal function can make or break you hormonally. Protecting these tiny regulators is therefore essential to stay well, but when you are going through ongoing stress they can start to become stressed themselves and adrenal fatigue can develop.

There are four stages of adrenal fatigue that I see in patients. Some know they are exhausted but take their symptoms lightly, with no idea how far down the path of adrenal fatigue they've traveled; others are desperate to find out how burned out they are. Here's how to tell which stage you're at (fingers crossed it's not too far):

- **Stage 1, compensation phase:** I call this the "compensation phase" because when you are at the beginning of adrenal fatigue, your cortisol rises in an attempt to compensate for the stressor that affects you. At this point, our mother hormone DHEA also endures the stressors well. Signs that you're in the "compensation phase" include mild tiredness when you wake up (even after a good night's sleep). Patients I see at this stage quite often say, "I need a coffee to start my day, otherwise I can't get going." Tiredness can also hit mid-afternoon, where again you start to crave sugar or need a coffee to keep you going. These quick fixes help you compensate for the fact that your adrenals are not working optimally. Reversing stress at this stage will reverse symptoms, but many people think this is "normal" and just keep going.

- **Stage 2, tired but wired:** If stress continues in this state, your endocrine system starts to tire. It diverts energy into making cortisol and, as such, your production of DHEA can drop. This is the point when I most commonly see patients. They know something is not right because that combination of high cortisol but low DHEA makes them feel anxious, and some even develop panic attacks. Libido can also lower. If you're affected you'll find it difficult to wake up in the morning, and have trouble getting to sleep or staying asleep at night, even though you're tired because your mind is whirring. You may also wake up hungry at about 3–5 a.m., as your blood-sugar level drops. You're probably easily irritated, feeling more cold as the thyroid gland becomes affected and possibly gaining weight around the middle, despite exercising. Oh, and the local barista knows you by name as you need so many cups of coffee to get through the entire day.

- **Stage 3, pre-burnout:** Both cortisol and DHEA levels have now plunged because the body is using up the DHEA levels to deal with the ongoing stress and the adrenals can no longer secrete high levels of cortisol to compensate. Normally cortisol must be high in the morning to wake us; the fact that it's not means at this stage most of my patients really have a hard time getting out of bed and continually reset the alarm to snooze. Your enthusiasm for life and your libido might fall. Your immunity is also likely to suffer, so you could find that you're picking up more minor bugs. Insomnia is likely as are other mental symptoms, such as anxiety and even depression. This can go on for a long period—and many of us still just think we're living a normal busy life and power through with the help of coffee, sugar and, probably, by now, the odd energy drink. But remember: every time you feel anxious or tired, this is a cry for help from the adrenal glands. They don't want more coffee or something sweet in a can; they need TLC. Otherwise, you will progress to stage 4.
- **Stage 4, burnout:** The cortisol levels continue to drop, flatlining throughout the day. This is a sign that the body is in real trouble. Your body can no longer manufacture stress hormones—all the symptoms of pre-burnout occur but they're magnified. In some patients it gets so bad they can't even get out of bed or do the things they love. At this point, they often visit their doctor and are prescribed antidepressants, which don't treat the cause at all. If you stay in this burnout phase for more than a year, I've found it can take years to restore optimal adrenal function. It's really important to seek help before this point.

How to test adrenal function

I believe the gold standard to check for adrenal fatigue is salivary hormone testing. Four saliva samples are taken—upon waking, at lunch, mid-afternoon and midnight, measuring the levels of DHEA and cortisol. However, there is a test that can check adrenal health you can do at home. It isn't as accurate as saliva testing, but alongside listening to your body and paying attention to any of the symptoms I describe above, it can reveal if your adrenals need some support.

- **The pupillary light reflex test:** Get a flashlight and stand in front of a mirror in a dark room. Shine the flashlight from the side at a 45-degree angle into one eye, being careful not to shine the flashlight directly in your eye. Monitor what happens to your pupils over the next 30 seconds.
  - » If your pupil becomes smaller for more than 20 seconds, this is healthy.
  - » If your pupil contracts, but then starts to pulse, slightly dilating then contracting, this indicates slightly low adrenal function. You need to stop trying to do everything and get some balance.
  - » If it starts to pulse after 5 seconds, this is a sign that your adrenals are under a moderate amount of pressure. Stress is taking its toll on your body and it's important that you take some clear steps to manage it.
  - » If there is immediate pulsation and dilation, your adrenals are exhausted. You are well underway to adrenal fatigue and are most definitely aging faster than the average person. Take a vacation immediately, doctor's orders, then it's essential that you follow the tips in this plan, but I'd also definitely suggest seeing a naturopathic doctor or integrative medical professional, as your adrenals need some extra support.

You can buy supplements of DHEA online or in health stores, but I don't recommend you try it without supervision from an appropriate medical professional. Remember, your body converts DHEA into estrogen and testosterone, but the amount we produce is highly individual. As such, you need someone to monitor your DHEA usage to ensure you don't end up misbalancing another hormone while trying to correct this one. Instead, to reduce risk of a faster DHEA decline, work on protecting your adrenal glands to keep them functioning optimally for as long as possible by reducing stress; tackle any sleep problems as poor sleep also lowers DHEA (see Chapter 6). Maintain a healthy weight, exercise, be happy and get out into the sunlight (wearing an adequate SPF, of course), as all of these things also help your body produce DHEA.

hGh—human growth hormone (and its friend IGF-1)

Made in the pituitary gland, hGh helps stimulate your body to grow, repair and build. It's very important if you want to arrest a lot of the overall physical decline of aging and stay strong and mobile as you age. As for the skin, low hGh is very firmly associated with poor skin repair and increased skin sagging. The lower its levels fall, the faster your face does too. However, hGh also works hand in hand with a second hormone, IGF-1, which is produced alongside it. This combination specifically stimulates collagen production. IGF-1 also helps stimulate production of new skin cells that give skin its youthful glow.

But the hGh/IGF-1 combination also fights aging in another way. Remember those receptor holes in the cells I mentioned? IGF-1 fits into the same one as the hormone insulin. As you'll see shortly, insulin is one of the most aging hormones your body can be exposed to—if IGF-1 is already in the holes, insulin can't get in and trigger damage.

As with all of the youth-boosting hormones, the production of hGh falls naturally as we age. Because of its important role in tissue growth, we produce our highest levels in our teens and 20s when we make it both when awake and asleep. As you leave your 20s, though, levels start to decline; by the age of 30 some people won't be making any at all during the day. By your 60s and 70s, you produce a fifth of the amount you did in your 20s.[5]

Signs you might be low in hGh:

- Aches and pains in the joints or muscles
- Dull, dry skin
- Fatigue
- Loose, sagging skin
- Low libido
- Muscle weakness/loss of strength
- Poor sleep
- Rapid wrinkling
- Slow wound healing
- Slower recovery from exercise
- Thinning hair
- Weaker bones
- Weight gain—especially around the middle

If you search online, you'll see people offering hGh supplements for sale; you can also have it administered by injection in some clinics around the US and the UK—please don't be tempted. What happens if you start supplementing with this powerful hormone has not yet been adequately studied and it could be potentially dangerous—just because something naturally appears in the body, it doesn't mean we should always have extremely high levels of it throughout life. Instead, you should try to boost your levels naturally, working with your body rather than overpowering it. I'll discuss two supplements that do this a little later, but as a general dietary rule, eating enough protein helps ensure adequate hGh production. Also, eat low glycemic index meals and avoid sugars and excess carbohydrate snacking. Two other very pleasant ways to raise your levels are getting enough sleep—remember, during sleep is the main time when hGh is primarily produced, particularly once we get older—and also having more sex; the author of that study I mentioned that associates youthful looks with a good sex life believes this happens because sex increases hGh levels.

The other way to raise hGh is via exercise—particularly weight training using heavy weights and with few rests in between sets, or short high-intensity cardiovascular workouts. When it comes to promoting positive hormonal reactions, the intensity of exercise is more important than the duration—that's good news to me as exercise has always been a challenge for me because of the time involved, but knowing that only 20 minutes a day can produce a result makes it far easier to achieve. I'll talk about the type of exercise I think is specifically anti-aging in Chapter 6—for now, just remember, when it comes to hGh, you want to be snoozing, moving and feeling frisky.

Thyroid hormones

Produced by the thyroid gland at the front of your throat in response to signals from the pituitary gland in the brain, thyroid hormones are involved in controlling almost every area of the body—including the skin. The thyroid can go wrong in two main ways: it can speed up, a problem called hyperthyroidism; or it can slow down, known as hypothyroidism. This second issue is a problem I'm seeing more and more in my clinic in women aged 30 and over—and is also the type most associated with premature aging. If the thyroid starts to slow down, it will show in the skin as dryness and skin thinning, but also as eye bags and puffiness—these appear as a side-effect of fluid retention that can be triggered when the thyroid slows.

Again, thyroid function naturally slows with age, but the thyroid is also extremely vulnerable to environmental damage. I refer to it as the delicate gland because it is so easily affected by things going on around us. Many chemicals we're exposed to each day affect the thyroid—it's been shown, for example, that some areas of the UK with fluoridated water have twice the incidence of hypothyroidism.[6] Smoking is also extremely damaging to the thyroid gland.

Your adrenal glands also support your thyroid, so the rising incidence of adrenal fatigue is also playing a role in many of the cases of hypothyroidism that I'm seeing.

Symptoms that your thyroid might be slowing down:

- Anxiety
- Cold hands and feet
- Dry bumpy skin on the back of the arms
- Dry thinning skin on the face
- Fatigue
- Foggy thinking
- Hair loss or thinning
- Insomnia
- Menstrual irregularities
- Thinning eyebrows
- Weight gain that won't shift no matter how little you eat

The temperature test

This home test can indicate if your thyroid is underperforming. If you're premenopausal, do it on the second or third day of your period, as temperature rises toward mid-cycle. If you're postmenopausal, it won't matter so much when you do the test as it's ovulation that triggers the temperature rise, and once your periods have stopped you are no longer ovulating.

- Place a mercury thermometer, shaken and ready to use, next to your bed.
- As soon as you wake up, before you do anything, place it under your armpit and leave it there for 10 minutes. Lie very still—you're trying to get a reading of your true core temperature at the time of the day when it should be at its lowest. Moving around will raise this.
- Measure it for four days. If the temperature is below normal—97.7–98.2°F (36.5–36.8°C)—for two days running, or if it averages less than 97.3°F (36.3°C) across the four days, it's likely that you are hypothyroid and you should seek further advice.

If you seek help from your primary care physician, however, be prepared to be told there is nothing wrong with you. To determine if your thyroid is underperforming, levels of two substances will be measured: thyroid stimulating hormone (TSH), which is produced by the brain and makes the thyroid work, and a hormone called T4 (thyroxine), which is the main hormone secreted into the blood by the thyroid. A high level of TSH and a low level of T4 signify clear hypothyroidism, and in this case, you will be prescribed a drug form of thyroxine to rebalance your levels. If you have high TSH and normal T4, you are at risk of developing a thyroid problem, and so, you'll be monitored more often. If your reading is "normal," though, don't assume your thyroid is performing well. For starters, orthodox testing classes an abnormal TSH level as over 4.5 mU/L. Personally, I see patients with evidence that their thyroid function as less than optimum when their TSH reaches over 2.0 mU/L.

On top of this, though, there's another problem that orthodox thyroid testing doesn't even take into consideration. There are actually two types of thyroid hormone: T4 and a second, more active hormone called T3 (triiodothyronine) that is created from T4. However, some people can't make that conversion or, if they do convert T3, it can't all enter their cells because the receptors are blocked by those "dirty hormones" I mentioned. This means that even though their numbers seem normal, these people aren't making the active hormone their thyroid actually needs to perform. It's estimated about 15 percent of sufferers of hypothyroid problems have "Low T3 Syndrome."[7] In my clinical practice I see a clear correlation between adrenal fatigue and thyroid issues, but it has also been linked to lowered selenium levels in the diet as the body needs selenium to convert T4 to T3. The foods we eat absorb selenium from the soil in which they grow or, in the case of livestock, from any contained within the grain-based feed they consume. However, the problem is that in much of the world, selenium levels in soil are now depleted. A food produced in one part of the country might therefore have levels 100 times higher (or lower) than that grown in another. Still, saying that, eating more selenium-rich foods is still the best way to maximize your levels—try nuts, seeds, shellfish, eggs and brown rice. Insufficient iodine in the diet is also a problem, so add natural sources, such as sea vegetables, fish, shellfish and a little iodized salt. Reversing inflammation (yes, our old friend again) and decreasing exposure to the "dirty hormones" will also help protect your thyroid.

THE AGE FASTER CREW

These are the hormones more likely to make you look and feel older if they become imbalanced.

Insulin

Insulin's normal job is to balance blood-sugar levels in the body. It's released from the pancreas in response to the presence of glucose in the bloodstream and it shuttles that glucose into the cells where it can be used for energy—or, if you produce more glucose than you need, it pushes any excess into your fat stores. The fact that insulin is an essential hormone can be seen by what happens when the insulin system breaks down—the development of type 1 or type 2 diabetes.

The problem is that as we age our cells become less sensitive to insulin; they effectively stop listening to the signals from the levels we produce. This problem is called insulin resistance, and it's strongly linked to premature aging, most seriously because it raises the risk of diseases of aging, such as heart disease and type 2 diabetes, but it also affects the skin. If your body doesn't respond to insulin, glucose, which is a sugar, is left circulating in the bloodstream for longer than it should. This can trigger the process of glycation and the subsequent production of AGEs (see page 72). Remember, glycation is a major cause of skin aging and also causes inflammation.

Insulin resistance or insensitivity can also imbalance many of the other hormones you need for healthy aging, as insulin can be involved in their production or transport around the body. All of them can be negatively affected if your body stops listening to the signals of insulin. If you want to stay young, you must avoid developing insulin resistance.

Signs of insulin resistance:

• Weight gain, especially around the stomach
• Tiredness after meals—particularly those containing high levels of sugar or refined carbohydrates
• Sugar cravings
• High blood pressure, high triglycerides and a low level of the good form of cholesterol, HDL

These signs generally only occur when the condition is fairly advanced, though—much of the time insulin resistance goes unnoticed.

The most common cause of insulin resistance is high levels of sugar (from sweet sources and refined carbohydrates) in the diet—the quicker foods turn to glucose in the body, the more sugar is produced and the more insulin your pancreas releases to combat that. In time, though, your body gets used to those insulin surges and simply stops listening.

There's not a direct test for insulin resistance, but high levels of glucose in the system generally indicate it's present. The most commonly used test involves checking levels of blood glucose in the system when you're in a fasted state—if this is between 5.5–6.9 mmol/L, you are classed as being in a pre-diabetic state and should urgently take steps to try to reverse this situation. The CDC reports that a third of Americans—86 million adults—have prediabetes. And in the UK, it's estimated that 7 million people are pre-diabetic.[8] You can get this test if you have signs and symptoms of type 2 diabetes or a family history. If you are over 40 years old, testing may be part of the standard preventative tests given, though this may vary with providers. It's available for anyone else at pharmacies such as Walgreens and CVS Minute Clinics for a small fee.

There is, however, also a secondary test called a Glucose Tolerance Test, which picks up problems earlier, before glucose levels in the blood start to rise significantly—and therefore before they start to increase the signs of aging. This compares your glucose levels before you drink a sugary drink and 1–2 hours after. If your insulin performance is normal, your blood-sugar levels should be roughly the same in both tests. If, however, your sugar level is still high in that second test, your insulin system is impaired in some way. I also suggest saliva testing for insulin levels as, again, it can help pick up problems early.

If you do have high insulin levels, adopting a low GI-based diet (like the Age-Reversing Eating Plan on page 204) will help prevent a sudden rise in blood sugar that triggers problems. Increase your intake of omega-3 fats, which directly fight insulin resistance by making the cell more permeable to the hormone, and most definitely carry out all the steps in the Inflammation-Fighting CCP Plan on page 95—inflammation increases insulin levels. Sleeping well also helps control insulin levels; in a study by Leiden University Medical Center in the Netherlands, even just one night of poor sleep led to poorer glucose control and higher insulin levels the next day.[9] Exercise also helps make the cells more sensitive to insulin. Again, both are covered in Chapter 6.

Cortisol

Released when you are under stress, cortisol is another of the hormones produced by the adrenal glands. Its normal jobs include vital functions, such as shuttling sugar into the muscles during stress and shutting off the inflammatory response that occurs at this time. Released as and when we need it, cortisol is an extremely helpful hormone to the body—and actually fights aging because it switches off inflammation. The problem is that our stressful lifestyles mean our bodies are now often in a state of near constant cortisol production.

Cortisol is the Goldilocks of hormones—your levels have to be just right. Too low and you develop adrenal fatigue (which triggers aging), too high and you'll also age faster as cortisol loves to damage skin, attacking it up to 10 times faster than any other tissue in the body. Every person I see with a high cortisol level has thinner skin than their peers—or is on the way to developing it. As I'll explain in the next chapter, decline in bone levels are now also strongly linked with facial aging—and just like the skin, bones also thin when cortisol levels are high.

Signs of high cortisol levels:

- Fatigue
- Finding it hard to wake in the morning
- Increased lines and wrinkles
- Loss of enthusiasm
- Low libido
- Poor immunity
- Sudden energy late at night
- Sugar and caffeine cravings
- Thinning skin
- Weight gain around the middle

The number one way to lower cortisol is to lower stress levels, but it will also help to keep your weight under control. Cortisol levels are higher in those carrying extra pounds, particularly those who carry that fat around the middle. You should also sleep well—like insulin, just one night of poor sleep raises cortisol levels the next day. Exercise also helps reduce cortisol levels.

There are many other hormones specifically involved with generalized aging of the body, notably testosterone, melatonin and progesterone. I haven't focused in detail on those here as I don't want you to feel as if you're taking a biology exam rather than reading a beauty book, but trying to ensure that the levels of these hormones are optimized is also vital. The problem is modern life does like to prevent this from happening.

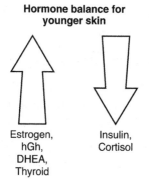

Hormone balance for younger skin

Estrogen, hGh, DHEA, Thyroid

Insulin, Cortisol

IT'S TIME TO TALK DIRTY

I've just discussed some of the reasons why specific hormones might become imbalanced. These, as well as inflammation and poor gut health, are factors that affect every single one of my patients (and their hormone levels) to some extent. However, absolutely the biggest factor unbalancing our hormones today is chemical exposure.

Every day we're exposed to thousands of chemicals. They enter our lungs via the air, our bodies via drinking water and the food we eat, or our skin via the cosmetics and toiletries we use, and they even appear in the clothes we wear or the furniture we sit on. It's been estimated, for example, that we are exposed to up to 515 chemicals each day from our beauty routine alone.[10] In one recent trial, monitoring chemical exposure with the use of absorbent wristbands, a group of 30 random volunteers were shown to be exposed to 49 of 1,182 of what researchers called "chemicals of concern" within just 30 days[11] and, shockingly, when experts at the Environmental Working Group sampled the umbilical cords of 10 newborn babies, they found traces of more than 200 chemicals.[12]

While, of course, not every chemical is harmful and not every chemical impacts your hormone levels, there are a number of chemicals that have been linked to hormonal disruption in the body. I touched on them briefly when I spoke about the role of xenoestrogens and how they might imbalance estrogen, and fluoride and its potential links with thyroid problems. But this group of chemicals known as endocrine disruptors have also been shown to impact adrenal hormones and testosterone. There are many of them, but some you could be commonly exposed to include:

- **Bisphenol-A (BPA):** Found in plastic packaging, including water bottles, drink containers, yogurt containers and microwave packaging, BPA also forms the lining inside of tin cans. This is believed to mimic reproductive hormones, including estrogen.
- **Dioxins:** These are by-products of industry but we mainly encounter them via the food supply, as they collect in animal

fat. They interfere with the ways that hormones, particularly the reproductive hormones, communicate.

- **Phthalates:** Used to soften plastic, these are commonly found in plastic food containers and plastic wrap. They also appear in beauty products as they are used in fragrance. Again, they are suspected to affect the reproductive hormones—for example, women with the highest levels of phthalates in their system were two-and-a-half times more likely to report disinterest in sex than those with lower levels as reported in a study by the University of Rochester.[13]

- **Mercury:** We are most commonly exposed to mercury via the food we eat, specifically oily fish. Mercury has been shown to impact the hormonal system in five different ways, including changing concentrations of hormones, binding to testosterone and altering levels of the enzymes needed to create hormones such as estrogen and testosterone. It's been shown to affect thyroid hormones, adrenal hormones and the reproductive hormones.

- **Arsenic:** Found in drinking water and foods—particularly rice. Arsenic has been shown to interfere with the genes that control the production of stress hormones, such as cortisol, and also affect estrogen receptors and the signals they send out.

The exact impact these chemicals, and the hormonal disruption they cause, are having directly on our bodies is only just being teased out via research, but on the very day I started writing this book, January 28, 2015, a new study came out from the Washington University School of Medicine in St. Louis. It examined 1,442 menopausal women and analyzed their exposure to 111 man-made chemicals either believed to be involved in hormone disruption or that are known to lodge in the body for a long period of time.[14] The study found that the women with the highest levels in their system had reached menopause two to four years earlier than those with the lowest levels. And while the researchers were clear to say that doesn't prove cause, it certainly suggests to me that these are not things we want to put into our bodies if we want to age more slowly—or age well.

Now you might say, "But I only use a tiny amount of moisturizer, how can it harm me?" or, "But there are laws in place that regulate the use of chemicals that mean we're only exposed to tiny amounts," and that is true, but there's now also emerging evidence that the chemical cocktail we're exposed to each day might also have a cumulative effect on our hormones. Safety officials are right in their calculations that one chemical in a small dose might not have a harmful effect on your body, but exposing your system to eight or nine chemicals in mini doses together may combine to have a different, more harmful effect.[15] As such, attempting to reduce your chemical load is an extremely important step in trying to get control of your hormones and reverse the signs of aging.

THE HORMONE-BALANCING CCP PLAN

This plan falls last in the book as many of the root causes of hormone imbalance can be eliminated if you look after the gut and fight inflammation. Why is this? For starters, hormones are partly eliminated via the gut, so if your digestive system is not working correctly, there are many ways that this system gets interrupted. If you're not pooping once a day, for example, you won't eliminate hormones satisfactorily and as they sit in the bowel, a case of leaky gut gives them the chance to escape back into the system through those enlarged tight junctions (see page 26). If you have imbalanced gut bacteria, they too join the party—estrogen, for example, can be reactivated by some harmful types of gut bacteria, which then tricks your body into allowing it back into the system at a point when its work should have been done. If your gut isn't healthy, you will end up with "dirty hormones" circulating the system—it's like Hotel California: they check in, but they never leave.

Inflammation can also trigger hormonal imbalances. It's associated with higher levels of estrogen, and it can aggravate thyroid conditions, worsen insulin resistance and lead to excessive cortisol release. Simply lowering inflammation in the body can therefore modulate a lot of hormonal issues.

If you have tried those plans, though, and are still getting the symptoms associated with any specific hormonal imbalance, then it's time to turn to the advice contained in the following pages. As before, I'd suggest following the steps in order, taking the Clear steps first, then moving to Correct and Protect. Again, spend two weeks following the Clear steps to allow the benefits to take effect in your system, then move on to the Correct steps for one or two weeks, followed by the Protect plan. Again, remember the Power Up suggestions are optional but will really help boost your results, particularly if you think that you're suffering from problems related to a particular hormone.

Clear

This part of the plan aims to remove the main elements that can help play a role in disrupting hormone imbalance—one of them you've probably already done via the other plans, the other might take a bit more of a lifestyle makeover.

1) Get rid of the Ultimate Agers

Yes, gluten, dairy, sugar and alcohol can all play a role in hormonal imbalances too. Here's exactly why:

- **Gluten:** There's some evidence that this might interfere with hormone levels—notably a reproductive hormone called pro-lactin—in people who are sensitive to it. If you are intolerant to gluten, the inflammatory response this creates also causes overproduction of cortisol.
- **Dairy:** Milk, particularly full-fat milk, and any products made from it can contain estrogen and contribute to your body's estrogenic load.
- **Sugar:** I briefly spoke about how this might be linked to higher rates of insulin production, but sugar can also trigger cortisol

release, as when blood sugar plummets (as is it will after a high-sugar meal), the body releases cortisol. On top of this, sugar can cause fat to collect in the liver and you need a well-functioning liver to detoxify hormones.

- **Alcohol:** If the liver is trying to remove alcohol from your body, some of its energy for handling hormones is diverted. Alcohol can also directly impact levels of many of the aging hormones too. Most alcoholic drinks are high GI, raising insulin levels very quickly; alcohol also directly raises levels of estrogen and cortisol, and lowers levels of hGh.

2) Chemical-proof your life

It's impossible to avoid every single endocrine disruptor you could be exposed to in life, but you can reduce your exposure with the following tips:

- Reduce your intake of processed foods and choose unpackaged products where possible. This will reduce your exposure to any of the chemicals contained within plastics and cans.
- Choose lean meats and remove obvious fat, which reduces exposure to any chemicals stored in animal fats. Choose your oily fish carefully, picking smaller fish such as sardines and anchovies.
- Follow the organic eating rules on page 41 to reduce pesticide exposure.
- Fit a water filter to reduce exposure to any chemicals in tap water.
- When you cook rice, rinse it first and cook it in lots of water so you can discard the cooking water, then rinse again (rather than having it absorb into the rice).
- Choose chemical-free cleaning products.
- Pick cosmetics and toiletries with short ingredient lists, mostly natural ingredients, and that as far as possible state they are paraben- or phthalate-free.

POWER UP

Try calcium d-glucarate. We naturally produce this in our bodies and it's involved in the process of detoxification. When your liver decides to send a substance it classes as harmful out of your system, it does so by packaging it up into a compound called a glucuronide. This is sent to the bowel, where, if all goes well, it leaves your system the next time you visit the bathroom. This process, however, can be interrupted by a few things, including poor gut health and high levels of an enzyme called beta-glucuronide. Calcium d-glucarate reduces production of beta-glucuronide, helping ensure the dirty hormones pass out of your system successfully. Take 500–1,000 mg daily if you want to rev up your natural detoxification system. However, because it can speed up liver metabolism, if you're on prescription medication, particularly statins, the contraceptive pill or antidepressants, such as diazepam, speak to your doctor before using calcium d-glucarate.

Correct

In this part of the plan, you're specifically trying to rebalance any hormones you believe might be out of balance—but you're aiming to do it in ways that work with your body.

1) Do the big three

Ensure you're sleeping well, dealing with stress and exercising correctly—exactly how you do all of these things will be discussed in Chapter 6. While these factors are important for good all-around health, they are extremely effective ways to help naturally balance hormones—remember: it takes just one night of poor sleep to imbalance some hormones; it can take the same to help restore harmony again.

2) Consider having a hormone profile test

Because many hormonal imbalances can manifest in similar symptoms, it can be hard to identify exactly which are causing your problems without professional analysis. Also, hormones interrelate—if your levels of estrogen are low, for example, you won't produce as much human growth hormone (hGh). Increase estrogen too high and you'll prevent testosterone and progesterone from working adequately. Trying to just correct one hormone in isolation therefore can cause side effects among other forms of these vital messengers.

In some circumstances your doctor may measure hormone levels—if, for example, you are a woman approaching menopause, or if you have the symptoms of type 2 diabetes or a thyroid disorder. However, often you won't be tested or, if you are, you will only be told you have a clear problem if you fit within specific medical ranges (see page 124). This doesn't mean that your fluctuating hormone levels are not having an impact on your body—or that altering them is not going to improve your health, your symptoms or your skin. In this case you may need a private hormonal profile test, which a naturopathic doctor or other integrated medical professional can order for you. Remember, as I've already mentioned, a saliva and/or urine test will pick up problems before a blood test.

If you do find levels of a particular hormone are imbalanced, you have a few options: you can alter your lifestyle in some of the ways I suggest for the individual hormones above; in some cases, you can correct the hormone levels via medication if needed or you can use bio-identical hormones, which are natural forms of hormone replacement that it's claimed your body better responds to. These can be given in supplement form or used topically. I would, however, suggest looking into some of the many natural supplements that can also help balance hormonal levels. Some of those I regularly recommend are:

- **Maca:** From Peru, this is one of the adaptogen family of herbs, which work to balance your body. This makes it particularly good in conjunction with the reproductive hormones as it won't raise levels that don't need alteration. It's also anti-inflammatory.

In studies, maca has been linked with favorable estrogen and testosterone levels, thus preserving your youthful hormones,[16] and is shown to help tackle symptoms of menopause caused by hormonal fluctuation.[17] There's not a set dose for maca—how much you use depends on your weight, age and how your body reacts to it. Start with 3 g daily of a powder, adding a little more if you don't get effects. The maximum dose consumed should be 9 g daily.

- **Chasteberry extract:** Also known as agnus castus, this helps balance progesterone levels. If you regularly suffer from PMS-based symptoms, such as mood swings and anxiety, you might be sensitive to lowered progesterone. Try 200 mg daily.

- **Black cohosh:** This is a member of the buttercup family and acts like an estrogen in the body, helping block the receptors in which the "dirty hormones" (see page 114) can collect. The recommended daily dose is 6.5 mg of extract (which is equivalent to 29.25–55.25 mg of black cohosh). It's extremely important to only buy a black cohosh product directly from a naturopathic doctor, trusted integrative medical professional or a brand that is marked with the THR mark, which guarantees purity. Cases of liver damage have been associated with contaminants in unregulated black cohosh products.

- **Relora:** This is a mixture of two herbs called magnolia and phellodendron, which are used traditionally to reduce stress and anxiety and lower cortisol. In studies, people taking it for four weeks lowered their cortisol level by 18 percent and their mood also significantly improved.[18] Because it takes the stress off the adrenal glands, Relora also helps naturally support DHEA production. Rhodiola is another great herb for helping stabilize adrenal function, as it's incredible for helping with stress.

- **DIM:** Also known as diindolylmethane, this is naturally found in cruciferous vegetables, such as cabbage. It helps your body detoxify and rebalance estrogen levels. It's particularly helpful for anyone who thinks they may be suffering from estrogen dominance. Try 100–300 mg daily.

- **L'Arginine:** This amino acid helps raise production of hGh (see page 121)—in fact, in trials at Syracuse University, it was found to double the amount produced in the body.[19] The recommended dose is 5–9 g a day: don't take more because it can cause problems such as bloating or stomach upsets if you overdo it, and it's counterproductive to upset the gut while helping your hormones.
- **Fenugreek:** This hard-working herb acts on both insulin and hGh, so you get a double-whammy positive effect. However, its ability to increase insulin sensitivity and decrease insulin resistance is what puts it on my dream team. It's so powerful that it's even shown positive results in lowering glucose levels in those with diabetes (ask your doctor before using it for that and don't combine with diabetic medication or warfarin). A good starting dose of those with only mild insulin imbalances is 2.5 g twice a day.
- **Bittermelon:** This strong antioxidant helps support insulin in that it naturally helps lower blood-sugar levels. Extracted from a gourd, its claim to fame (over and above its insulin-balancing ability) is that it's believed to be the most bitter fruit or vegetable you can eat—thankfully you don't get the taste if you consume it as a supplement. It's believed to act in three different ways that combine to lower glucose levels in the body. Try 100–200 mg daily of a product stating that it is standardized to 10 percent bitters, which shows it contains the right amount to be effective. Do not use if pregnant.

Protect

In this final step you're introducing changes that help support the main hormone-balancing and detoxification systems of the body.

1) Increase the green detoxifiers

Vegetables from the cruciferous family, which include cabbage, cauliflower, broccoli, Brussels sprouts and kale, are particularly good at helping your body excrete estrogen successfully. The magic ingredients within them are called indoles, which form compounds that bind to estrogens and carry them out of the system. These are the same substances that you find in DIM (see page 137), but in a lower dose.

2) Look after your liver

You've already started doing this by cutting down on sugar, fat and alcohol, and increasing detoxifiers, but also fill your diet with natural liver-supporting foods, such as onions, garlic and turmeric, and herbs like rosemary, thyme, oregano and sage. Avocado is also a food your liver loves. It helps the body produce glutathione, which helps the liver work more effectively. Finally, the regular use of castor oil packs (see the instructions on page 64) will give the liver a boost.

> **POWER UP**
> The herb milk thistle is like the superhero of liver support. It converts into glutathione, it acts as an antioxidant and an anti-inflammatory, and it helps regenerate liver cells. I recommend 200–250 mg of a standardized extract (ideally choose a brand that states it contains 80–85 percent silymarin) three times daily.

3) Sweat

Sweat at least three times a week in something like a sauna, steam room or via exercise. The skin is the body's largest organ of elimination and it's believed that regular sweating helps detoxify the body of many toxins, including heavy metals such as mercury. Heat is also calming to the body, making a regular sauna session a great stress fighter—but it also boosts the skin by opening and unclogging the pores and raising circulation. Try it and just see how much your skin glows afterward.

4) Add isoflavones

Found in foods such as fermented soy, chickpeas, alfalfa and peanuts, isoflavones act like natural estrogens in your body—in a good way. They will lock into cells' receptors in the same way normal estrogen does and trick your body into thinking your estrogen levels are higher than they are. Unlike the "dirty hormones," though, this is a natural and harm-free mimicry that can help counteract some of the natural fall in estrogen that occurs with age. On top of this, if an isoflavone is blocking the receptor, those "dirty hormones" can't get in to do harm. Don't overdo your isoflavone consumption—some is good; more may not be better. Just a small portion or two a day is enough to gently support your body.

5) Eat the rainbow

The more antioxidants you have in your diet, the more protected your body is going to be from those environmental chemicals that you can't control. The more colorful your diet, the more antioxidants it will contain. Try to eat the rainbow every day:

- **White:** Apples, eggplant, bamboo shoots, bean sprouts, cauliflower, chicory, daikon radish, fennel, leeks, zucchini, mushrooms, onions, pears, radish, shallots, spring onions, white cabbage.
- **Orange:** Apricots, butternut squash, cantaloupe, carrots, clementines, mangos, oranges, papaya, peaches, persimmon, pumpkin, satsumas, sweet potato, tangerines.
- **Red:** Cranberries, goji berries, grapes, pomegranates, raspberries, red peppers, rhubarb, strawberries, tomatoes, watermelon.
- **Yellow:** Bananas, corn, galia melon, lemons, pineapple.
- **Blue/purple:** Acai, beets, blackberries, blackcurrants, blueberries, plums, red cabbage.

- **Green:** Alfalfa, artichokes, arugula, asparagus, avocado, fava beans, broccoli, Brussels sprouts, celery, zucchinis, cucumbers, green beans, green peppers, kale, limes, lettuce, okra, peas, runner beans, savoy cabbage, seaweed, spinach, spring greens, Swiss chard, Tuscan kale, watercress.

So there you have it; I hope you can now see how hormonal fluctuations, whether they are natural or caused by the chemicals around us, can speed up the rate at which you age, and that if your hormones go south, so will the rest of you! But I also hope you now see how much you can do to potentially slow that decline.

Now let's move on to the fun bit of anti-aging: the true beauty side of things: skincare, treatments and make-up, and how to use these to the best advantage to care for your skin and turn back time.

CHAPTER 5

THE BEAUTY PRESCRIPTION

So far I've only talked about how you fight premature aging from within, but once you've taken care of the inside, what you put on your skin and what treatments you decide to partake in regularly are the final determining factor as to how your skin looks and feels on the outside. They are absolutely vital to reversing the signs of aging and protecting your skin against future damage; marry the right treatments inside and out, and you'll have the perfect fit that busts aging now and in the years to come.

Of course if you're standing in the pharmacy, department store, beauty salon or spa looking at row after row of products or an entire menu of treatments all claiming to turn back time, it can be hard to know what exactly your skin regimen should consist of. The same confusion can occur when you walk into a health store looking at row after row of skin supplements, all claiming they too have the latest, greatest solution to beating aging. Well this is where I come in.

Over the years I have examined the scientific data behind hundreds of beauty products, treatments and supplements—and seen how they behave in the body and affect my own skin and that of my patients, and I have identified what I believe are the most effective products and treatments out there. Shortly I'll talk you through exactly what they are and how to use them—but first, here's a crash course in skin 101. If you understand your skin better, you'll also understand how to get the best out of it.

SKIN DEEP

Measuring an area of 16–22 sq ft (1.5–2 sq m), the skin is the body's largest organ and also the fastest growing one. Each inch of your skin contains 19 million separate cells, and every single day the body sheds and replenishes 30,000–40,000 of those. It's constantly in motion. But it's also constantly under attack, particularly the skin on your face, and to some extent, your neck and hands. Think about it: these are the only areas of your body that are constantly exposed to the outside world. It's no surprise, therefore, that these are the areas where the signs of aging appear first.

The skin is made up of three main layers, each of which has a different role in keeping it healthy and youthful. In young, healthy skin, all of these functions behave optimally, but as we age, things start to slow or change, altering the way the skin acts and looks. This triggers the natural development of signs of aging, such as lines, wrinkles, pigmentation, dull, rough skin, and a mottled or uneven skin tone. This natural body slowdown is known as intrinsic aging, and it happens to everyone. It begins internally in our 20s, starts to show externally for the first time in our 30s or 40s, and nothing in our beauty arsenal so far can stop it completely—although you can help slow and reverse it a little. That might sound like very bad news, but it's not—because intrinsic aging alone actually accounts for very little of the aging we see on our skin.

What ages us is exposure to external factors, such as sunlight, pollution, poor diet and inadequate hydration. This is called extrinsic aging and it's the main reason most of us age. Even though they occur internally in the body, all the reactions triggered by poor gut health, excessive inflammation or hormonal changes that I've been discussing throughout this book are also classified as extrinsic aging. When it comes to aging prematurely, extrinsic aging is what you need to prevent and fight against.

IS YOUR FACE OLDER THAN YOU ARE?

Of course to know if you're aging naturally or experiencing the accelerated aging we want to fight, you need to know what to expect as you age. As a general rule, this is what happens at various ages, although do remember that the more extrinsic aging factors, such as sun exposure, you expose your skin to, the earlier changes will occur:

- **25 or under:** At this age, the skin should look plump and youthful, your skin tone should be even and bright, and lines and wrinkles should be virtually non-existent—unless you have a very expressive face, in which case they might faintly appear around your smile lines, between the brows or across your forehead. One change you might notice is that your pores get a little larger, which is one of the first signs of lowering collagen levels.

- **25–35:** It's normal for some lines to appear by now—particularly under the eyes, off to the sides as so-called crow's feet, and the side of the mouth. The reason is the 10:10 rule—you lose about 10 percent of your collagen every 10 years, so every decade you'll start to notice a greater increase in wrinkles, lines and sagging skin. The good news is your skin tone should still be even, but you might start to notice that it looks a little duller and your skin might feel drier.

- **35–45:** The face starts to lose shape now as you start to lose fat that lies under the skin. Lines and wrinkles become more pronounced, particularly the marionette lines that run from the sides of the mouth to the chin, and nasolabial folds that run from the side of the nose to the mouth. Falling collagen levels also lead to a slight hooding of the eyelids and laxity on the face and neck. Your skin tone might lose some brightness as cell turnover slows down, but the skin texture should still be smooth. You will notice the skin start to feel drier and tighter. Annoyingly this can also be a prime trigger point for adult acne as hormone levels start to become imbalanced in the run up to menopause.

- **45–55:** Fat levels continue to fall, but as you approach and then pass menopause it's the drop in hormone levels that cause the majority of changes. The skin becomes considerably drier, and this alone makes it more likely to crease and wrinkle. As collagen loss speeds up, this accentuates the laxity that begins in your early 40s and jowls can appear as the face starts to sag. You could also notice your skin start to look a little more sallow as circulation becomes less effective.
- **55+:** By now the bone structure of the face has also changed, which adds to all of the above problems. The brows droop and the lips start to thin. Pigmentation cells can also start to behave erratically, which can trigger blotchy skin and the appearance of age spots.

Some of you will have read that and felt a little hopeless. We live in a society now where it's being seen as normal to iron out every sign of aging and, as such, reading about the above might fill some of you with dread. But remember: all of us age and we can't, and shouldn't, erase every aspect of that; features such as laughter lines and smile lines are a sign that you've lived a little, and that your life was filled with love, fun and happiness—you should be proud to show them off. You shouldn't want to fill or freeze every line on your face, but nor do you want your face filled with other lines not reflective of all those good times. Those are what we're aiming to reverse with the advice in this book!

This need for balance in your face is why I don't think face-freezing or filler injections reverse the signs of aging. It's true they have revolutionized the anti-aging industry, but to me they aren't the answer to fighting premature aging effectively. You can have as many jabs as you like but they won't change the texture of your skin or the pigmentation and skin tone it exhibits. Plus you get trapped into constantly having them redone to look "normal" and you can then fall into the trap of not remembering what is normal. This then leads to the type of overuse of injections that makes you look older, not younger. Don't get me wrong, I'm not saying "never use face freezers or fillers"—if you have a really, really deep furrow that bugs you then injectables are the only thing that will fix that, but to me that shiny forehead, shiny face, lifted, frozen or puffy look can make many people look older than they are, and that is definitely not youthful and definitely not what we're trying to achieve.

HOW THE FACE AGES: A LAYER-BY-LAYER GUIDE

The skin's layers

The epidermis

This is the outer layer of the skin and it's made up of two layers of cells. The uppermost layer is called the stratum corneum, which forms the skin's barrier—its job is to stop irritants from entering the skin and help ensure that oils and water that keep the skin plump and hydrated stay inside. The stratum corneum is also involved with keeping the skin hydrated. Cells within it draw water into the skin, while other cells degrade, causing the release of fatty acids and fatty substances called ceramides that keep the skin supple and moist.

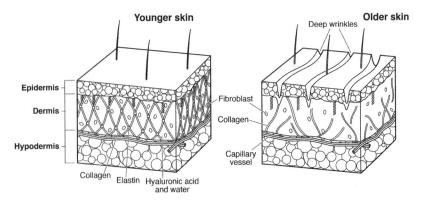

Considering they are effectively the skin you present to the world, it might surprise you to find that the cells that make up most of the stratum corneum are actually dead. New, healthy cells are produced lower down in the skin, which then migrate up to the surface and push those dead cells off the surface, a process called desquamation. In young skin, this process takes around 28 days, but as we get older the process slows down; by the time you're age 60 it can take almost twice that time for cells to be shed. This slowdown is why your skin looks duller as it ages—dead skin cells don't reflect light as effectively as the live ones do. Any buildup of dead cells can also lead to your skin looking and feeling slightly rougher as you age.

The second layer of the epidermis consists of cells called basal cells. These produce the new skin cells that populate the stratum corneum. Also found within the second layer of the epidermis are cells called melanocytes, which make the pigment melanin that determines your skin color. The more melanin you produce, the darker your skin. Melanin is also what causes your skin to tan if you go out into sunlight. As we get older, however, the melanocytes can become more erratic, releasing higher levels of pigment in certain areas—inflammation and hormonal imbalances can both worsen this. This can lead to the formation of age spots on the skin but also hyperpigmentation (see page 111).

The dermis

This is the middle layer of the skin and the thickest section. Within it you'll find the skin's nervous system, which controls what the skin feels in terms of temperature, pressure and pain. It's also where the sweat glands, hair follicles and sebaceous glands are located. Of these, when it comes to aging, it's the sebaceous glands that interest us most. These glands can be affected by a fall in estrogen and subsequent dominance of the male hormone androgen that trigger dryness and adult acne—a combination that increasingly I'm seeing develop in patients in their 40s and 50s.

The dermis is also where the collagen, elastin and hyaluronic acid are located within the skin. We hear these terms all the time in the beauty world, and you probably know that they are involved with how fast or slow you age, but do you know exactly what they are?

- **Collagen:** Collagen is a protein produced in the skin by cells called fibroblasts. It's responsible for supporting the skin's structure and keeping it firm and strong. In young skin the collagen fibers are packed tightly and actually as strong as steel. As we age, though, these fibers straighten and become more loosely entwined. This reduces firmness and increases the skin's ability to fold, crease and wrinkle. The amount of collagen you produce falls by about 10 percent per decade, and by the time you're age 60 you're unlikely to be making much new collagen at all. This makes it harder and harder to repair any damage that occurs.

- **Elastin:** Elastin, as the name might suggest, is the skin's elastic—it helps it spring back when you crease or bend it. As you get older, though, elastin begins to stiffen, and just like an old elastic band, it starts to slacken. The fibers also get thinner and longer with age. This stops the skin from snapping back, leading to wrinkles and facial sagging.

- **Hyaluronic acid:** This molecule appears in the base of the dermis and is one of a group of cell molecules called glycosaminoglycans (GAGs). The job of GAGs is to hydrate and cushion tissues within the body. Hyuralonic acid is excellent at its job—it can contain up to 1,000 times its own weight in water, so having enough in the body is key to plump, youthful-looking skin, but every day you use up about a third of your hyaluronic acid, which must then be replenished. Like so many processes in the body, though, the body's ability to do this decreases as we age and by the time we reach our mid-40s, we only make about half as much as we need. This contributes to drier skin, but as hyaluronic acid is also involved in the formation of collagen, it also contributes to how fast levels of this start to fall. As such, the dermis is where lines and wrinkles—the signs many of us associate most strongly with aging—begin.

Hypodermis

This third layer of the skin is made up of fat, which plumps up the skin, and the more of it you have, the younger your face looks. As we age, though, the amount of fat within the face begins to degrade— often because of damage from those extrinsic factors I discussed. In my experience people with Sugar Face (see page 71) also suffer a premature aging of the face caused by a lowering of the fat levels in the skin.

It used to be thought that all the fat on the face was the same and therefore was lost at the same rate, but it's been discovered that the fat is actually contained in 16 compartments around the face[1] and that these degrade at different rates, with the upper cheeks normally the first area affected. Stress particularly causes facial fat loss. In a study by leading UK plastic surgeon Dr. Rajiv Grover, some women lost up to 35 percent of their facial volume within just one year of a traumatic event, such as bereavement, unemployment or divorce.[2]

THE FACIAL BONES

These support the skin's structure, and recent research has discovered they play a fundamental role in how well we age. A study published in the journal *Plastic and Reconstructive Surgery* that looked at three groups of people, aged 20–40, 41–64 and over 65, found clearly that changes that occur to the bones as we get older explain a lot of what happens to the face as we age.[3] For example, our eye sockets become wider and longer, which could contribute to eye bags, eye lines and dark circles; the bones of the middle face change and the nose widens, which can worsen marionette lines; while the angles of the jaw substantially alter, contributing to sagging of the lower face that also worsens wrinkles on the neck. In women, the biggest changes occur between the ages of 41–64; in men it starts a little later. As such it makes sense to also try to protect your bone health as you age with good nutrition, healthy exercise and lowered levels of inflammation.

PAMPER YOURSELF PRETTY

It's time to get on to the fun bit—lotions, potions, creams and gels. The perfect skincare plan should aim to reverse and protect against as many of the above changes as possible—that's quite a complex mission, and I hope you'll see that just rubbing in a little moisturizer now and again probably isn't going to cut it! I therefore suggest you take a three-pronged approach to anti-aging skincare that's similar to the plans we've been using throughout this book in that it aims to Clear, Correct and Protect against factors aging the skin.

THE SKINCARE CCP PLAN

Clear

Clearing the skin means cleansing the skin. The most important role of cleansing is to get rid of excess oil, make-up and any kind of dirt or pollutant. If these sit on the skin, they clog the pores, increasing the risk of pore enlargement, acne and dullness. During cleansing you also gently resurface the skin, giving the cells the chance to turn over more quickly than they would normally, which allows younger cells underneath the chance to appear. You also create a clean skin free of congestion and dead skin cells that help the next products you use penetrate the skin. Done well, cleansing can actually help you create a younger-looking and acting skin—so, here are the three steps to cleansing well:

Step 1

If you wear eye make-up, remove this first. Use a gentle, but effective eye make-up remover that doesn't require you scrubbing at your face to get results. Using a remover that doesn't dissolve make-up well, requiring you to rub hard, will stretch and age the skin. The secret to using make-up remover is to soak a cotton ball well, then hold it against your eyes for a few moments to let the active ingredients get to work dissolving the shadow or mascara. Then, gently wipe away your products.

Note: if your eyes sting when you use remover, swap brands. This is not normal and will actually trigger a mild inflammatory response— you've worked so hard to try to lower inflammation in your body, so avoid using products that trigger it.

Step 2

Turn your attention to cleansing the rest of your face. I suggest to most of my clients that they use a cleanser containing one of two ingredients: glycolic acid or salicylic acid. Both of these work in the same way, by dissolving the bonds that hold dead skin cells on to the surface of the stratum corneum. By doing this, the cells are shed sooner. Not only does this instantly reveal the younger, brighter cells underneath, it also triggers the cells of the basal layer to start production again, helping naturally rev up cell turnover. They can also lighten areas of pigmentation.

Glycolic acid is made from sugar. It's one of a family of skincare ingredients called alpha-hydroxy acids (AHAs). The others in the family include lactic acid from milk, and malic acid from apples and pears. Of the AHAs, I prefer glycolic as it has the most established usage and research behind it. Glycolic is particularly good for those with more mature skin as it stimulates the production of collagen and elastin. I also recommend it to anyone suffering from Wine Face (see page 69) or Sugar Face (see page 71) as it's very good at helping eliminate fine, feathery lines that often develop if you overdo alcohol or sugar.

Salicylic acid is an ingredient found in the bark of the white willow tree. It's a beta-hydroxy acid (BHA). The main difference between beta-hydroxy and alpha-hydroxy acids is that BHAs are oil soluble. This makes salicylic acid better if you have oily skin. It's also particularly good for people who have acne or skin that tends to break out as it has anti-microbial properties and is anti-inflammatory (salicylic acid is also the ingredient that aspirin is based upon). Anyone suffering from Dairy Face (see page 65) will also benefit from a salicylic acid.

You can choose a product that uses just one of these acids, or one that combines smaller amounts of both. The exception to this rule is if you have very sensitive skin, which can react to glycolic or salicylic acids. In that case I'd suggest using a cleanser with one of two ingredients that work wonderfully on more sensitive skin. *Chamomilla recutita* (*matricaria*) extract is a potent antioxidant that helps reduce irritability during cleansing, providing a calming effect to the skin. Asiaticoside asiatic acid (*Centella asiatica*) is another potent antioxidant that helps stimulate collagen production, and it also helps support and keep the capillaries strong, so it is particularly good for people with rosacea.

You should cleanse twice a day using your cleanser and a soft cloth and water—and two to three times a week, depending on how sensitive your skin is, try adding a Clarisonic brush. I love my Clarisonic. If you haven't come across these yet, they are rotating cleansing brushes that gently jiggle the skin, opening the pores just wide enough that they release dirt from deep down inside. In one study, using a Clarisonic was found to remove six times more make-up than cleansing manually.[4] In fact it's so effective that the reason I don't suggest using it every day is that it can actually clean and exfoliate the skin *too* well, which can either make it dry, or cause it to overcompensate and make more oil. On days you aren't using the brush, just use your fingers to massage in the cleanser. In both cases, though, always move upward, outward and around. Just as with your eye make-up remover, you never want to pull the skin downward or rub too hard. Finally, only use lukewarm water. Hot water can be very drying to the skin and may encourage the formation of broken blood vessels.

Cleansing as described above uses the perfect combination of ingredients and techniques that both remove pollutants from the skin and trigger regular gentle exfoliation. Exfoliation is great for the skin, but if you use this approach you don't need to use any other scrubs as part of your plan.

Correct

When the skin is clean, it's primed and ready to receive ingredients that help correct damage. Here are the ones I suggest you try:

1) Start with a skin-boosting serum

Serums target specific problems in the skin. I have clinically researched a number of cutting-edge ingredients commonly used in the formulation, and because these ingredients are so good at creating youthful skin, I have implemented them with my patients accordingly. Depending on their skin type and their skincare goals, I might prescribe patients just one of these or a combination, which can create a great synergy of ingredients. To help you decide which is best for you, though, here are details on what each of my favorites can do.

- **Vitamin C:** A stabilized form of this called l-ascorbic acid is absolutely the most important antioxidant when it comes to reversing aging. Anyone in my clinic who wants younger skin goes on vitamin C—it's a skin superhero that's good for everything. It helps with collagen synthesis, it's anti-inflammatory and it helps the skin heal from everyday environmental attacks. If lines, wrinkles and thinning skin are your main concern, it should definitely be part of your routine. Vitamin C also inhibits the enzyme tyrosinase, which causes hyperpigmentation and age spots. You might wonder why you shouldn't just take it orally to get these effects—well, according to a report in the *Journal of Cosmetic Dermatology*, you actually receive 20–40 times more vitamin C when applied topically than if you take it as a supplement.[5] Remember, though, vitamin C is destroyed by exposure to light and air. Products containing vitamin C should be in a dark bottle and ideally have a pump-style dispenser rather than an open lid.
- **Co-enzyme Q10:** This is a vitamin-like substance that the body makes in the liver—generally, it's used to produce energy within the cells of the body, and this also holds true for its role in the skin. It helps aid cell production, so it's particularly good if

you feel the brightness of your skin is suffering. Q10 also helps protect against UV damage, reduces levels of collagen-degrading enzymes in the body and has been clearly shown to fight crow's feet.[6] We naturally produce less Q10 after age 30 but, on top of this, both the contraceptive pill and statins further lower Q10 levels in the body. If you are using either of these, Co-enzyme Q10 might be a good addition to your routine.

- **Plant stem cells:** Plant stem cells are taken from meristem, tissue found in plants where growth and rejuvenation occur. Because of their role in growth, the molecules in plant stem cells help the skin repair. They also have an antioxidant activity even stronger than that of vitamin C. These cells enhance collagen production and inhibit the process of glycation that makes collagen hard and stiff. Plant stem cells are perfect for those with Sugar Face (see page 71). I particularly recommend extracts *Gardenia jasmonoides* (from the gardenia plant, which is renowned for collagen synthesis) and *Leontopodium alpinum* (from edelweiss, which is particularly effective in the eye area).

- **Marine collagen:** Marine collagen is absorbed up to 1.5 times more efficiently than other collagens. Marine collagen has the smallest molecular size and weight among all collagens and has been shown to stimulate cellular immune responses that not only help prevent the skin from UV-induced water loss but also increase collagen synthesis.[7]

- **Fucowhite (*Ascophyllum nodosum*):** This brown algae is one of the most researched algae among the academic community. Fucowhite has been shown to increase skin clarity and decrease skin pigmentation.

- ***Centella asiatica:*** Also known as Gotu Kola, *Centella asiatica* has anti-inflammatory properties. It increases hydration and helps soothe and repair dry, red, irritated skin.[8] I have used this skin remedy with patients for decades.

- **Green tea:** Well known for its internal health benefits, topical green tea is particularly anti-inflammatory and so might be good for those with acne and rosacea. It's also been shown to inhibit the MMP enzymes that degrade collagen and elastin in the skin.[9] Green tea might also be particularly good if you are concerned specifically about the texture of your skin. Women using a green tea–based cream reduced skin roughness in as little as 30 days in one trial.[10]

- **Pycnogenol:** Another powerful anti-inflammatory substance, pycnogenol binds to the collagen and elastin within skin, helping increase their strength and protect them against damage. It also increases the skin's natural protection against UV rays, stopping aging at its source. Finally, it's a good choice for women with acne. In one study, 75 percent of women using it topically reported improvements in their breakouts.[11]

2) Apply a cream or serum containing hyaluronic acid

I briefly mentioned this before (see page 148), so you may remember this is the main molecule involved in ensuring the skin stays hydrated. Levels fall as we age, but using it topically helps counteract that. That alone makes it worthy of inclusion in any skincare regime, but I particularly like to use it right now because applying hyaluronic on top of antioxidants helps push them deep into the skin where they can work effectively.

3) Moisturize

The job of any moisturizer is to add hydration to the skin's uppermost layer. When this is well hydrated, more water is attracted into the skin, and less is shed from the upper layers. The added layer of moisture that moisturizer provides also increases the amount of light reflected from the skin's uppermost layer—that's why skin can look instantly healthier when you apply moisturizer.

There are many types of moisturizer with different active ingredients, but you might find one product I suggest my patients start to use very unusual, and that is snail mucus. This has been very popular in countries like Korea for some time and has now made its way into Western skincare. It may sound like a strange thing for me to suggest, but in a world where we're bombarded with chemicals, I try to keep the skincare I suggest simple, safe and effective, and this fits the bill for me. It's particularly good for those with dry skin, whether that's younger skin where dryness is the main concern, or older skin that gets drier as hormone levels fall.

The story behind its discovery is very interesting. Snail farmers in Chile noticed their hands were becoming smooth and soft and that if they cut themselves they healed very quickly. This caused scientists to become interested. They started to analyze the mucus and slime that snails emit to protect their skin and shell, and they discovered that one ingredient in this, called *Helix aspersa Müller*, contained a mix of ingredients commonly found in cosmetics, including glycolic acid, hyaluronic acid, collagen and elastin. It also contains peptides, which are active proteins that allow the cells to communicate with each other. In this case the peptides stimulate the skin cells to produce more elastin and more collagen. Not surprisingly cosmetic companies then decided it would be a good ingredient for skincare.

Retin-A (tretinoin) and Retinols

Each night replace your moisturizer with a product containing Retin-A, also known as tretinoin or a retinol. These are the gold standard in anti-aging ingredients. Derived from vitamin A, they increase cell turnover, fade fine lines and wrinkles and effectively communicate with your skin cells, suggesting they behave like the younger, healthier cells they once were. Both are also impressive antioxidants. The difference between them is in their strength: Retin-A is stronger and must be prescribed by a dermatologist, doctor or other qualified skincare practitioner; retinols are milder and more tolerable.

Many studies have been published on Retin-A and retinols. I won't go into them all; instead I'll just tell you about the latest one I came across in my research.[12] This, unusually, focused on retinols—most use Retin-A—and what it explored is exactly what happened to sun-damaged skin when people used a formulation of 0.1 percent retinol for a year. They found crow's feet reduced by 44 percent, pigmentation decreased by 84 percent and skin produced more collagen and hyaluronic acid.

Despite this compelling evidence for their use, more is not better. Both are very potent and overuse can upset the skin leading to reddening and flaking. Let your skin get used to them by starting off using them just three times a week— say Monday, Wednesday and Friday—for a few weeks. If your skin feels okay, then start using them daily—always avoid using them under the eyes though. Also both Retin-A and retinols are damaged by UV rays and therefore should only be used at night. This also means any product you buy containing them should be in a sealed opaque container. As with vitamin C, never buy a retinol-based product in a jar with a lid that can be removed.

Another ingredient I'm interested in is topical probiotics. There's a lot of research going on regarding the use of these in skincare at the moment, and it seems they are very healthy to the cellular activity and help boost the skin's protective mechanism against stress and environmental damage. They also help reinforce the skin's barrier, and some forms have been shown to fight the bacteria that causes acne.[13] If you don't like the idea of the snail mucus, or have more sensitive or oily skin, then I would suggest using moisturizers that integrate probiotics to their formulations instead.[13] In my Treatment Mask No 1, I have included a special prebiotic ingredient to support the skin's micobiome.

As you get older, skincare needs to work a little harder, and the ingredient I suggest to help with this is plant stem cells. These work as fantastically in moisturizers as they do in serums. Remember, these cells are taken from some of the hardiest botanicals on the planet, like the Swiss Uttwiler Spätlauber apple, which is famed because it can be stored for weeks without starting to shrivel, or the Alpine rose, which grows 10,500 ft (3,200 m) above sea level and yet protects itself beautifully against the high levels of UV radiation found at that altitude. I think the discovery of stem cells is amazing science. The idea that the extract of a genetically long-living plant could be applied to human skin and stimulate your own cells to work harder is incredible. I use plant stems cells in my treatments all the time.

4) Use an eye cream
The skin under the eye is the thinnest in the body and the first area many of us see the signs of aging. You absolutely must treat it and I particularly like to use creams containing growth factors in this area. Growth factors help stimulate fibroblasts, the cells that make collagen. They're naturally produced after injury and stimulate the skin to repair. I particularly like products with copper tripeptide as this has good evidence behind its action and is naturally found in the skin. Copper tripeptides help repair wrinkles and reduce the appearance of dark circles, resetting your skin's DNA around the eyes to a youthful glow. When you apply an eye cream, be extremely gentle—don't rub and, again, don't drag the skin downward. Apply a couple of tiny dabs at the point where your eye hollow starts, then use your little finger to gentle smooth these into the skin. The natural movement of the eyes when you blink, smile or speak will then help it migrate to where it needs to go.

Facial Massage: The One-Minute Beauty Boost

If you want an inexpensive, super-simple, extra speedy way to boost your skin regime, incorporating facial massage into your daily routine is it. You can use the following routine as you apply your moisturizer morning and night to help improve the skin's circulation and tighten the facial muscles. As an extra bonus, it helps the products absorb effectively too.

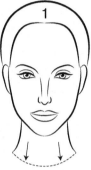

1) Swipe your moisturizer over your face as normal, making sure you also cover your neck (it always amazes me how many of my patients stop their skincare at their chin).

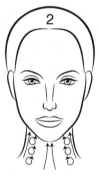

2) Use your right palm to massage the moisturizer into the left-hand side of your neck, moving upward in mini circles. Repeat on the other side with the other hand, then smooth up the middle of the neck with both hands together.

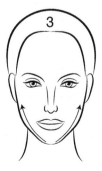

3) Move to your chin and holding your hands underneath, as if you were praying, use your fingertips to smooth the skin upward along the jawline and to the ears. Lift your fingers off the skin and repeat again. Do this three to four times. You'll immediately feel tension in your jaw start to release.

4) Keep working on the outer sides of the face, but now use the fingers on both hands to stroke upward from the level of your earlobes to your hairline.

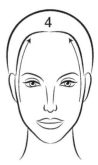

5) Move to the center of your face. Using the tips of two fingers, stroke outward from the sides of the nose, under your cheekbone out to your hairline. Now, using those same two fingers, gently press five to six times along the top of the cheekbone, under the eye moving sideways from nose to hairline.

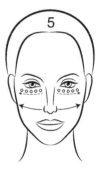

6) Place two fingers of each hand side by side between your brows at just above brow height. Massage upward toward the hairline. When you reach the top, lift your fingers off the skin then return to the brows a little further toward the sides of your face. Repeat until you've smoothed your whole forehead.

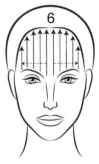

7) Finish by stroking quickly from the middle of the face outward, working down in lines from the top of the forehead down toward the chin. Your whole face should now feel energized. If any moisturizer is left to rub in, do that using gentle upward movements.

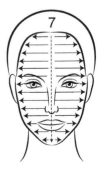

Protect

When it comes to topical skincare, there's one absolute must-use for protecting the skin: sunscreen. UV damage is the number one cause of extrinsic aging, and it's estimated to account for 80 percent of all premature aging. UV rays trigger the destruction of collagen and elastin, they cause inflammation, and they can contribute to excessive pigmentation and poor skin tone.

There are two types of UV rays. The first is UVA, which accounts for the majority of those in the sunlight that reaches us. These rays penetrate deep into the dermis of the skin and trigger the production of free radicals. These are also the rays that switch on melanin production and the potential hyperpigmentation that can come with it. The second type of rays are called UVB, and these damage the DNA of skin cells. The biggest concern associated with UVB rays is that they have the potential to trigger skin cancer.

Every single day, you need to use a broad spectrum SPF 50 on the skin to protect against both these types of UV ray. Sunscreen can be mineral and chemical based. Each works in slightly different ways. Chemical sunscreens absorb the UV rays and then scatter them across the skin's surface, preventing them from penetrating inside where they can cause harm. Mineral sunscreens, which tend to be the whiter products, including ingredients such as zinc oxide or titanium dioxide, create a reflective layer that simply bounces the rays away from the skin before they do harm.

I don't feel either is any better or worse, but some people do find they react to chemical sunscreens and so should switch to a mineral-based brand. Whatever you use, though, should be applied every two hours if you're going to be in the sun for any length of time.

Personally I also wear sunglasses most of the time—even if the day is quite cloudy. A good pair of sunglasses conforming to US Food and Drug Administration Standards will effectively screen out UV rays, minimizing damage that contributes to crow's feet and crepey eyelids, but that also damages and ages the cells within the eyes themselves. Some companies now mark these with what they call an E-SPF—

Eye Sun Protection Factor. This indicates their level of protection—as with sunscreen, go for the highest E-SPF you can, which is a 50.

The routine at a glance

Morning:
- Cleanse
- Apply antioxidants
- Apply hyaluronic acid
- Apply moisturizer and SPF

Evening:
- Cleanse (2–3 times a week using the Clarisonic brush)
- Apply antioxidants
- Apply hyaluronic acid
- Apply retinols
- Apply eye cream

If you're on a budget, that routine might look a bit expensive, but most of the ingredients I discuss can be found in drug stores in relatively inexpensive ranges. However, if you want to just focus on the essentials, they would be to cleanse—use a simple oil-free cleanser with salicylic acid, which will cleanse the skin well but also help exfoliation—then use an antioxidant serum and SPF. You could also tailor the routine to your age or skin type: if you don't have dry skin, it's okay to leave out the hyaluronic acid; those in their 20s can get away without a specific eye cream; and if you don't have wrinkles, skin scarring, pigmentation or acne, then you might not yet need a retinol.

Five Skincare Products Best Avoided

While I think the products on page 169 are the best products to use, if you find a product that works for your skin then please, keep using it. However, there are a few products or ingredients that I'd prefer you steered clear of.

1) **Facial oils:** The skin likes to live in balance—if you apply oil to it externally it gets a message that it doesn't need to produce oils of its own. This means your skin can actually start to dry out as you use

them. Oil can initially make the skin feel good, but that doesn't mean it's giving it any long-term support.

2) **Creamy cleansers:** Many people with dry skin use these as they don't like the way other cleansers leave their skin feeling—however, I don't care for them. I find they can build up a layer on the skin that can stop your second layer of products from working as effectively.

3) **Petroleum-based products:** Some moisturizers use petroleum, but I find it quite clogging to the skin, and it can trigger breakouts. I also feel that occlusion can block the skin's cellular communication, meaning it just won't perform the way it should.

4) **Chemical-filled products:** There's a lot of junk in some products, and I think anything that uses a lot of chemicals is best avoided. I'd prefer you not to use products that contain parabens (a type of preservative), phthalates (contained in fragrances), dyes and colors, perfumes or sodium laurel sulphate. These chemicals can enter your bloodstream and cause changes in the hormone balance, which stresses the skin.

5) **Facial wipes:** These can contain an ingredient called methylisothiazolinone (MI) that many dermatologists are now linking to skin reactions. It's a preservative put in the cloths to prevent bacteria growth, but in some people it can cause contact dermatitis, which causes the skin to go red, itch and blister. Many companies are now removing MI, so check labels if you like to use wipes to make sure your brand doesn't contain it. It can also be found in some skin washes and moisturizers.

POWER UP: Treatments for the skin

Using the products I describe above will counteract daily damage and help your body stimulate its own age-fighting systems to help tackle aging from within, but if you want further help, having regular professional skin treatments and/or taking supplements that help boost the skin's anti-aging capabilities can give you the Power Up you need.

The treatments to try

While not everyone needs professional skin treatments, if you have already suffered many signs of digest-aging, or really want to significantly try to reverse your skin age, they will achieve more than just using topical skincare ever can. These are the ones I recommend:

Medical skin needling: A small roller studded with tiny needles is run gently over the face. This causes controlled damage to the surface of the skin, triggering an inflammatory response that causes the fibroblasts to boost their production of collagen. It's an excellent way to tackle fine lines, stretch marks, pigmentation and acne scars. Now it might surprise you to see me recommending something that *causes* inflammation to the skin here—I'm even surprised myself sometimes—but after medical needling, your skin can produce up to 400 percent more collagen.[14] This is a good example of how controlled inflammation can help the body. However, saying that, you shouldn't start medical needling until after you have completed the Gut-Balancing CCP Plan (see page 37) and ideally followed all the inflammation advice in Chapter 3. That will ensure your anti-inflammatory system is working effectively and will be able to switch off the inflammation the treatment generates once healing has occurred.

You can use needling on the face, the hands and the décolletage, but I think the best results come on the face. I recommend six treatments, six weeks apart. There is some downtime—your skin will look red immediately after treatment. The skin is far more sun sensitive after a medical needling treatment, so you absolutely must use SPF 50 from then on. If you want to witness a treatment, you can take a look at *the goop lab* on Netflix. In the "The Health-Span Plan" episode, you can watch me give a treatment to Gwyneth Paltrow.

You can now buy skin rollers online to use at home, and they will have some effect—albeit a limited one. To get an actual reaction that induces the formation of collagen, you need needles about 1.5 mm long, but those are far too long to use safely on your own skin and must only ever be used by a professional. If you want to try needling yourself, stick to rollers with needles 0.3 mm or under and use them at night a few times a week.

LED treatments: This came from research on NASA astronauts. NASA had started using lights from LEDs to help plants grow in space and then wondered if it might aid cell renewal in astronauts too (they wanted to help preserve bone and muscle mass and trigger wounds to heal faster). Trials found that as well as doing this, it raised levels of collagen and elastin in the skin. After this became public knowledge, the beauty industry adopted the technology. You can use two different colors of light—red LED light is anti-inflammatory and used to treat wrinkles, while blue light has been shown to kill the bacteria that causes acne and can be used to control sebum production, close large pores and reduce oily skin.

An LED treatment is painless: the wands are simply held over the skin and the light naturally passes into the skin just like UV does from sunlight—but with a more positive effect. Gels with vitamins and botanicals are applied to the skin that help the light penetrate, and in a beauty-based example of symbiosis the light also helps these gels penetrate deeper too. You will see some benefits right away from an LED treatment, but I generally recommend five or six in a row.

Hyperbaric oxygen infusion: This uses oxygen blown over the face to help infuse topical treatments deeper into the skin. It was developed to deliver cancer medications deep into the skin but, just like with the NASA finding, the technology was then adopted by the beauty industry to make delivering skincare more effective. I use it to deliver a mixture of antioxidants, plant stem cells, growth factors and hyaluronic acid deep into the dermis where they can work optimally. I particularly like the fact that the results are immediate. I can treat one side of someone's face and they will visibly see a difference; saying that, though, to get a long-lasting result you will need around 10 treatments as an initial course and then a refresher treatment every couple of months.

Radio frequency: This is the best treatment for tightening and lifting. It heats the skin at a very deep level and this causes the collagen to contract, which makes the skin look and feel tighter and more lifted. It also helps promote collagen production and increases oxygen and nutrient availability to the cells so, even aside from the tightening, the skin looks amazing. Again you need a series of these. I recommend six sessions over a period of six weeks— thereafter you can maintain monthly treatments for the rest of the year. You repeat the course 12 months later.

Microdermabrasion and peels: Anything that helps with cell turnover will make the skin look fresher, younger and more revived, and peels and microdermabrasion do this wonderfully. They also shrink your pores, which often enlarge with age, and remove blackheads. They tackle pigmentation, balance uneven skin tone and improve skin thickness by stimulating collagen production. Each treatment works in slightly different ways to achieve these amazing results. Microdermabrasion uses a high-pressure jet to lightly buff the skin with tiny crystals, while peels use concentrated forms of salicylic, glycolic or lactic acids to loosen the bonds between the skin cells and resurface things. Oh, and forget the days of old harsh peels where you had to take two weeks off work and the skin flaked off in sheets. Today's peels are gentle and have no downtime.

POWER UP: Supplements for the skin

Many of the antioxidants you apply to the skin can also be taken orally in supplement form, enhancing the benefits they create externally from the inside too. Here are the ones that are worthwhile:

Collagen: A specific type called hydrolyzed collagen contains extremely small collagen particles that increase the chance of them reaching the dermis. In trials, women taking 2.5 g of hydrolyzed collagen daily significantly reduced wrinkle depth (by at least 20 percent) in eight weeks.[15]

Alpha-lipoic acid: An extremely powerful antioxidant, it's rare as it is both fat and water soluble, meaning it can effectively enter many different parts of skin cells, fighting aging where it starts. Alpha-lipoic acid also fights inflammation, but its real power comes from the fact that it stops the stiffening of collagen fibers caused by sugar. Anyone with Sugar Face (see page 71) should definitely consider a supplement of alpha-lipoic acid. I recommend 80 mg a day.

Oral antioxidants: These will help effectively neutralize any free radicals in the system. While using them topically is fantastic for skin, taking them orally boosts results as they absorb into the bloodstream through the gut wall and reach the skin from the inside. As we age, the skin repair process slows down, and this added oral support gives it a much needed helping hand. Remember, though, it's important to take antioxidants in combination as they work together, so I suggest 1,000 mg vitamin C, 800 IU vitamin E and 5,000 IU vitamin A. When I give this combination to people, their skin becomes brighter and more hydrated in as little as four months. Note: if you are taking vitamin A for any other reason do not double up—levels of vitamin A over 10,000 IU a day can be toxic. Check any other supplements you are taking to make sure you aren't accidentally consuming too much. You can also try my Vitamin C Cocktail Powder, infused with true liposomal vitamin C, zinc, super berry antioxidants and phosphatidylcholine.

Hyaluronic acid: If you have dry skin, this supplement should be on your radar. Japanese research recently showed that women taking it showed a definite increase in hydration within as little as three weeks.[16] It's particularly good past the age of 40 when our ability to generate hyaluronic acid starts to fall significantly. Take 250 mg daily. You can also find this in my Beauty in a Bottle ingestible supplement (see page 291).

Fish oil: I've already mentioned how this fights stress and reduces inflammation, but the omega-3 fats in fish oil can also help hydrate skin. One 2005 study found that EPA, a type of omega-3 found primarily in fish oil, helps block the release of ultraviolet-induced enzymes that eat away at your skin's collagen, causing lines and sagging skin.[17] I recommend taking 1,000 mg a day of fish oil or omega-3 fatty acids.

MY LITTLE BLACK BOOK OF SECRETS

I'm often asked what's in my own personal skincare and make-up bags—and what I do to keep my skin well. I basically follow the routine I've discussed over the last pages, but with a few additions. I have also created my own line of supplements for the skin, which you can find on page 290.

The products I really love

- **My own line of products:** I spent time in Switzerland researching and creating my own product line. The items include the dream-team combination of ingredients that I now use on all the patients I treat. There are four products in the line right now—Dr Nigma Cleanser No1, Serum No1, Crème No1 moisturizer and Treatment Mask No1. After just one application, your skin will feel like it has drunk a liter of water. The moisturizer contains plant stem cells, marine collagen and natural growth factors that keep the skin feeling tight and bright. See page 290 for a list of authorized retailers.
  - » **Dr Nigma Cleanser No1:** Cleansers are very underrated but are one of the most important parts of any skincare regimen. I love my Cleanser No1, which is packed with volcanic ash and salicylic, glycolic and hyaluronic acids. This prepares your skin for applying and to optimally absorb the rest of your skincare products.
  - » **Dr Nigma Serum No1:** Packed with plant stem cells, hyaluronic acid, snail peptides and vitamin F, I recommend my Serum No1, which will instantly plump, tighten and protect the skin from UV exposure while also reducing overall skin inflammation.
  - » **Dr Nigma Crème No1:** The moisturizer I love the most is my Crème No1; it contains snow algae, soluble collagen, African birch bark and low molecular weight hyaluronic acid.

This cream is a game changer for deep hydration, brightening and repairing your skin from environmental pollution.

» **Dr Nigma Treatment Mask No1:** The best treatment mask is my own; I created this one-of-a-kind biocellulose sheet mask that acts like second skin infused with marine collagen, seaweed and algae extracts with prebiotic ingredients to support the skin microbiome, leaving the skin hydrated, plump, bright and lifted.

• **Heliocare:** For my daily sunscreen, I like Heliocare, which is especially good on sensitive skins that may react to other sunscreens. Not only does it use normal sunscreen ingredients, it also has its own combination of antioxidants called Fernblock that further prevents damage to skin cells.

I'm also a big fan of making my own beauty products from items you can find in your own kitchen. Here are six of my favorite recipes:

Traditional turmeric mask to dye for

I have used turmeric since I was a kid. My grandmother used to give me a paste of turmeric and honey when I had coughs and colds. She'd give it to me on a spoon and make me swallow it in one go. I used to cringe as a child, but my grandmother was on to something—now this amazing spice has everybody talking. When I use turmeric, it brings back warm memories of my grandmother. This is one spice I cannot live without.

Why is turmeric so cool and amazing? I can name a long list of turmeric's skin benefits: it's used to treat acne blemishes, blackheads, pigmentation on the skin, eczema and psoriasis. Turmeric is great for dry skin, and will help you slow down the aging process as it helps soften wrinkles. In India, turmeric has been added to cleansers and creams for years.

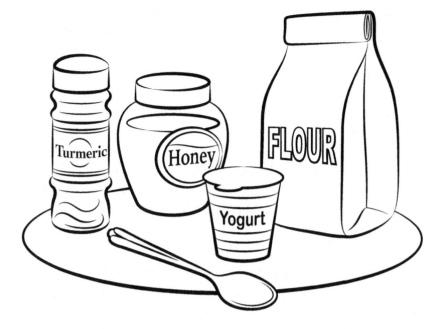

The following mask recipe can be used to help acne, pigmented skin, rough and dry skin and eczema flare-ups. It reduces inflammation and redness, and promotes skin healing. Use it three times a week if you have acne, acne scars or pigmentation. If you have normal skin with no inflammation, use this mask once a week as a skin brightener and tightener.

1 tbsp rice or chickpea flour
2 tsp turmeric powder
2 tsp natural yogurt
1 tsp runny honey
1 tsp grated lemon peel

1. Mix all the ingredients together to make a paste. This should be thin enough to spread easily on your face but thick enough to stick well. It shouldn't run down your skin.
2. Cleanse your skin with warm water and your daily cleanser.

3. Make sure your hair is away from your face and avoid wearing any clothing you love because turmeric's powerful dye is difficult to get off.

4. Apply to the entire face, including under the eyes, the neck and décolletage—use your fingers or a clean make-up brush.

5. Leave the mask on for 20 minutes and then rinse off with warm water.

6. Finish off your final rinse with cool water. After drying your skin, use a toner and/or make-up remover to remove any extra turmeric on the face. I'm not kidding about turmeric's powerful pigments: they can stain anything and everything, including the face.

Bye-bye acne treatment

I have two masks that I like to use if I ever suffer a blemish. The first is based on turmeric, as it's excellent at regulating the production of sebum on the skin, and I mix this with chamomile tea (chamomile is both antimicrobial and anti-inflammatory) and a little aloe vera juice, which can act against the bacteria that causes acne. This mask can also help fade any acne scars on the skin. The second mask uses a mix of cinnamon and honey. Like turmeric, cinnamon is a spice with many health-promoting properties, but here I use it because it has strong antimicrobial properties, which fight the bacteria that cause acne. Honey is also a natural antibiotic.

TURMERIC AND CHAMOMILE

2 tsp turmeric
1 chamomile tea bag
1 tsp aloe vera gel

1. Put the chamomile tea bag in a normal-sized mug and fill with about one-third of a cup of water. Brew for 3–5 minutes.

2. Remove the bag and add the turmeric and aloe vera. Mix into a paste.

3. Dab directly on to any blemishes or acne scars. Leave for 30 minutes then rinse off with lukewarm water.
4. Cleanse the skin as normal.

CINNAMON AND HONEY
2 tbsp runny honey
1 tbsp cinnamon

1. Mix the two together until it makes a smooth paste.
2. Apply directly to any spots or blemishes.
3. Leave on for 20 minutes, then rinse off with lukewarm water.
4. Cleanse the skin as normal.

Exfoliate, tighten and brighten

I came across this recipe during my university years when I couldn't afford to buy expensive over-the-counter scrubs. Even then I was trying not to put excessive chemicals on my face, so this had two benefits—it was cheap and natural. My friends and I would try different home treatments, but these were two of our favorites.

PAPAYA AND AVOCADO

We were ahead of our time with this—not only is papaya loaded with antioxidants, it's also packed full of alpha-hydroxy acid and of course the yogurt we used is a natural source of probiotics, one of the hottest trends in skincare right now. Honey has the ability to encourage moisture in the skin without triggering the buildup of excess oil, plus it's a natural skin lightener (as is lemon) so it is great for blemishes and dark spots. Avocado is also an extremely effective moisturizing agent and is therefore perfect for dry skin. Egg white tightens skin and is rich in vitamin A.

½ small ripe papaya
½ avocado
1 tsp runny honey
1 tsp fresh lemon juice
1 egg white
1 tbsp plain yogurt

1. Mix all the ingredients together in a large bowl.
2. Apply the mixture to clean skin and leave on for 5–8 minutes.
3. Rinse with warm water, then cool and pat dry.

DAIRY FACE MASK

I might not want you to eat yogurt for the sake of your skin, but it's good if you apply it topically. Add to egg white, which is rich in vitamin A, and you have another great mask.

¼ ripe avocado
1 egg yolk
1 tsp yogurt

1. Mash the avocado in a bowl.
2. Add the rest of the ingredients and mix into a smooth paste.
3. Apply to your face with your fingertips—remember: only go upward.
4. Leave for 15 minutes then rinse off with warm water.

Icing beauty

I created this trick when I was doing a breakfast morning TV show in Vancouver back in 2002 and I had to be up super early in the morning. Back then I wasn't a morning person but had to look and feel fresh, so I made this concoction one evening to plan for my morning routine, and over the years changed and fiddled around with the ingredients until—ta-dah—I came up with this. I use it when I have somewhere special to go or if I have been naughty eating gluten and have ended up with Gluten Face. It's also great to depuff the effects of Dairy Face.

Why ice and aloe is a great combination: ice reduces swelling and inflammation and it shrinks the capillaries, which diminishes the appearance of redness. Aloe vera helps kill bacteria that cause acne; it's moisturizing and anti-inflammatory, and it has astringent properties that help heal scars. Cucumbers are also good at soothing the skin.

½ cucumber
¾ cup aloe vera juice
½ tsp turmeric
¼ cup water

1. Blend the cucumber into a smooth paste using a food processor or blender, then mix with the aloe, turmeric and water.
2. Add the mix to an ice cube tray, filling as many holes as you can.
3. Freeze until they go hard.
4. Put the cubes in a bowl and place a towel around your neck to protect your clothing.
5. One at time, place a cube in a hanky or face cloth and then massage the ice cube evenly on your face until it melts. Don't put the ice directly on your face as this can damage the skin.
6. Repeat with a new cube; keep going until all the cubes are used up. This can take up to 40 minutes.
7. Keep your face frozen throughout (literally)—try to relax the muscles and not tense, even when you first apply the cubes.

CHARLOTTE TILBURY'S ANTI-AGING MAKE-UP TRICKS

I'm lucky enough to work with my good friend and expert make-up artist Charlotte Tilbury on various projects. When it comes to beauty and aging—and how to fight it—we both want to know the best and latest advice not only for ourselves but for our clients. Charlotte's clients include Sienna Miller, Kim Kardashian, Penelope Cruz and Kate Moss, and she really is among the world's top beauty experts. As such, I couldn't think of anyone I'd rather have advise you on the best ways to use the make-up you wear to help you look younger. So, I decided to quiz her on her absolute best age-reversing make-up tips.

Q: Let's start at the beginning—when it comes to foundation to help us look younger, what formulation should we be using?
Liquids. As you age, your skin dries out and powders can sometimes accentuate this by sitting in the lines and cracks, making you look older than you are. Be careful of cream foundations as, although they can be more moisturizing, they give heavier coverage that may sit in lines and pores. Instead, opt for a super-light liquid formulation that hydrates the skin and includes treatment and transforming ingredients such as hyaluronic acid, natural alternatives to retinol, or BioNymph peptides, which work in the deep layer of skin to boost collagen, reversing the appearance of wrinkles. You need luminous, breathable foundation textures that finish the skin with a dewy look, while also containing youth-boosting properties.

You can either apply foundation with a brush or your fingertips. A foundation brush will give you more coverage for targeting areas of, say, pigmentation or uneven skin tone; fingertips create a more natural look. Your fingertips are warm, which warms up the texture of foundation making it more malleable and easier to blend into the skin, thereby creating lighter coverage. If you have dry skin, heavy coverage can highlight any cracked or uneven skin tone. Instead, build up application to create a thin base using your fingertips. Skin that is dry can also appear more lackluster and dull, so painting back the luminosity into the skin is really important. Look for foundations and concealers that contain light reflectors, which scatter light across the face, giving a natural-looking glow.

If you decide to finish with a powder, be careful. Depending on your skin type, some powders can make you look dusty and accentuate an uneven skin surface. If I use powder, it is always a finely milled powder enriched with emollients, such as rose wax and almond oil, which are hydrating. For normal to combination skin types, only apply powder on the T-zone (forehead, nose and chin) and leave the cheeks dewy and full of glow to re-create a naturally youthful look. If you have oily skin, you may also want to apply the powder in a targeted way across the cheeks, but ensure you tap off the excess powder on the back of your hand before applying, as this will help you control how much you apply.

Q: What's the most common aging mistake people make when choosing their shade of foundation?
When they match the foundation to the back of their hand, because it's really rare that it matches the face. Instead, apply a line of foundation from the jaw down to your neck, and in good, natural daylight check in a mirror to ensure the shade matches both skin tones. The best shade will disappear into the skin, rather than create a tide mark, and cover imperfections.

Other aging mistakes:

- **Pale skin:** Avoid shades that are too pink because, while you might think they add color, they can in fact make your skin look flat and lifeless. A dewy, well-defined facial framework has the appearance of youth. A foundation with a yellow base can, in fact, be more flattering, as it naturally returns color and vitality to the face while still looking natural.
- **Darker skins:** Avoid shades that are lighter than your natural skin tone, as this can make you look gray and ashy, dulling the skin tone. You can in fact reverse the visible age of your skin with the correct foundation shade: choose a warm-toned shade instead that brings color back into the face, while softening the

appearance of lines and pores. Avoid going darker than your natural skin tone as, again, this will drain all your best features and make it harder to contour and accentuate.

Q: Is there a make-up trick to help soften fine lines and wrinkles?
You can't create a beautiful painting without a beautiful canvas. This is how I think about the link between a skincare regime and make-up application. I never start a make-up look without applying a moisturizing boost containing hyaluronic acid, rosehip oil and vitamin E to prepare the skin.

Q: Let's talk camouflage. What's your best tip for concealing under-eye shadows that often worsen as we age?
Choose a concealer with the right tone and texture. You want something creamy enough to hydrate and not look cakey, but with enough pigments to conceal. If you have really dark circles under the eyes, first apply a full coverage, peachy colored concealer to cancel out the darkness. Then trace over this with a retoucher pen to correct the color and match your natural skin tone, and finally apply a light-reflecting concealer. Light reflectors are great for the under-eye area as they combat discoloration, soft-focus lines and imperfections by bouncing light away from the problem area. They can correct the appearance of a sunken under-eye hollow too.

Q: If you don't have model cheekbones and a defined jaw, can we correct this? Also, as you age your nose and chin grow as well. Is there something we can do to correct this with make-up?
Facial contouring is like make-up magic, but many women are afraid of attempting it because they don't want to go wrong. Contouring the facial framework is one of the most fabulous tricks used by make-up artists and is easy for everyone to re-create at home once you know how. You too can contour out a new jawline, create killer cheekbones, slim and trim your nose and overall balance the framework of your face to highlight your best features.

To create the ultimate facial contour: follow the hollow

Look in the mirror, suck in your cheeks and literally follow the hollow underneath your cheekbone: use a sculpting brush, which should be V-shaped, to allow more precision and control.

Apply a bronzing, contouring powder just under the cheekbones in the hollow—this starts from the top of the ear to the fleshy part of your cheek. Brush upward, starting under the apples of the cheeks and blend. Never forget to tap off the excess product on the back of your hand before applying, as this allows you to build up color and therefore have more control.

Once done, apply a highlighter, which is a lighter, sometimes shimmery, powder, right along the top of your cheekbones, just under the eye. Sweep outward and up along the bone, starting just past the center and ending at the outer corner, in a C-shape. Blend by brushing away at the outer edges of the highlighter. To make the contouring less severe and to enhance the youth in your cheeks, add a pop of blush on the apples of your cheeks to finish.

To define your nose

As you age, your nose continues to grow because it is made of cartilage, but you can use the power of contouring to slim and shorten the shape and size—an instant nose job without surgery.

Start by using a smaller make-up brush—I use an eyeshadow brush. Apply a line of bronzing powder down either side of the nose from the top to the bottom. To further enhance the illusion of a sculpted, thinner nose, then you can apply a soft, subtle highlighter shade down the center. This draws attention to the thinnest part of the nose, slimming it, and also creates a greater sense of relief for noses that are flat.

Another trick is a shading technique that I use for longer noses. I apply a touch of bronzing powder to the tip of the nose between the nostrils. Optically, it shortens the nose.

The youth-plumping illusion

Q: Plumped-up cheeks are a sign of youth, and using blush well can create a hint of these—but what should or shouldn't we do?

A common blusher mistake is applying it too low down on the cheek. This has the negative effect of dragging the face downward and taking attention away from the cheekbones. For youthful, full and sumptuous cheeks, use a blusher brush to apply color high up on top of the apples of the cheeks and blend outward toward the ear for a seamless, natural finish. Or use creamy blush formulations, which can give a dewy, youthful finish. Remember to apply at the highest part of your cheekbones, blend well and absolutely pick the right shade for your complexion—you don't want to look like Aunt Sally! To lift paler skin tones, choose a pop of soft rose pink that mimics the color your skin naturally becomes when you blush. Medium to olive skin tones really suit a peachy pink hue. For a darker complexion, opt for muted berry shades to enhance the cheeks.

Eyes

Q: As we age, brows shrink—how do you counteract that?

Brows thin as hair regrowth slows down. As such, full, handsome and lush brows are the epitome of youth. Many women make the mistake of over-plucking, which can be aging. The eyebrows are the pillars of the face and when well-groomed can give your entire face a lift. Use an eyebrow brush to comb the hairs upward, then fill in hairs with a brow pencil or powder, then apply highlighter under the brows for an instant lift. When you are shading, stay as close as possible to your natural hair color, or even a shade lighter. Overly dark brows can be very unforgiving and overbearing on an older face, and can drain color from the skin.

Depending on your face shape, plucking the arch slightly can give you an instant lift that opens up the eyes, but never overpluck. Ideally invest in getting your brows professionally done initially and then you can follow that line in the future at home.

Q: When choosing eyeshadows, which are the best/worst formulations and colors to choose if you are starting to get lines around the eyes?

Use finely milled powders that are enriched with oils, so they blend easily and glide over the lid—you don't want using eyeshadow to drag the delicate skin. Emollient-rich formulas also have the benefit of not dropping on to your under-eye area. Opt for neutral tones, such as chocolates, taupes, creams and bronzes because they flatter all skin tones and naturally enhance and define the eyes in a chic, sophisticated and elegant way. Avoid formulations that are too bright, metallic or heavy—these can really age you, making the surrounding skin look paler and duller.

Q: Lashes can also thin as we age and the hair follicles decrease in diameter. How can you plump them without getting spidery lashes?

So many women bypass using an eyelash curler but this can give you an instant eyelift. Lash curlers are like a push-up bra for the eyes. They may look like instruments of torture, but they really have the magical ability of opening up the eyes, which tend to sag as we age, again creating an anti-age optical illusion.

Once curled, layer several coats of mascara, ensuring you coat all lashes, especially the smaller ones on the inner and outer corners. This will open up, widen and brighten your eyes. Also don't forget the bottom lashes as these will frame your eyes and give you definition. To apply mascara well, start at the base of your lashes, brush upward and outward in a zig-zag motion from the inner corner of your eye, to the outer corner. This will instantly lengthen and elongate your eyes, creating that youthful Bambi look.

Q: After the age of 40, eyelids can start to droop at the outer corners. Are there any make-up tricks to lift and brighten the eyes?

Yes, you can use eyeshadow to cheat away drooping eyelids and contour the lids—I use similar principles to facial contouring to achieve this.

Instead of applying a wash of shadow across the socket, as you may normally do, try applying it slightly above and into the socket line to enhance the sense of relief of your lid. It creates the illusion that your eyelids have lifted. Follow the hollow of the eye socket the same way you do to contour your cheeks. Using an eyeshadow brush, apply a natural taupe brown color, similar to a bronzing shade, starting at the outer corner of the eye and following the eye socket hollow toward the inner corner of the eye.

A feline flick, where you extend your eyeliner out past the outside of your eye to simulate a cat's eye, can elongate the eyes and lift them upward. Using a creamy black pencil or a liquid liner, draw a thin line along your lash line from the inner corner of the eye and stop three-quarters of the way along. Next, to define the outer tip of your cat's eye, draw a dot ½ in (1 cm) from the outer corner of your eye, then continue the line to join the dot and fill in the rest of the line. Finish with mascara on your lashes.

Lips

Q: Lips get thinner as we age, but is there a way to cheat your way to a bigger pout without resorting to needles?
Luckily, this is nothing that a slick of lipstick cannot solve! As lips lose their fullness and become more and more lined, darker shades can be harder to wear as they can make lips appear smaller. However, it's also important to not go too pale as this can wash out the color in your entire face. I think the most flattering shades are those that are a couple of tones more intense than your natural lip color. Generally speaking, a tawny rose shade suits everyone and gives you a natural, fresh and youthful look because it is the perfect lip color balance; not too dark or pale.

Lip gloss can also be great to add volume. Many women think that it's for younger people, but it can really create the illusion of plumper lips, especially when applied in the center of the lips outward as it creates the illusion of fullness. It's important to look for a sophisticated formula that applies more like a lacquer than a super-shiny gloss.

Always line the lips first—this will stop lipstick from bleeding, and when applied to the outer edge of the lips will cheat your way to a fuller pout. For a natural look, choose a lip liner and lipstick that mimic the shade of your lips. Match the liner to the lipstick shade so that you are not left with a harsh outline.

*

Don't you feel younger already? Well there's another secret to truly reversing aging that I need to reveal—and that's the day-to-day things you can do that turn back time. This might be exercising effectively, sleeping better, fighting stress by changing the way you react to it—and, my favorite, creating a younger mindset that turns back time and makes every day a joy to live.

CHAPTER 6

LIVE AN AGE-REVERSING LIFE

Our bodies faces attacks daily from things that increase our susceptibility to accelerated aging—and while our exposure to these might be partly out of our control, I hope you've seen from the previous pages how much you can do to counteract any damage by eating the right foods, taking supplements and making some simple lifestyle changes. But there are some final ways to turn back the clock that I haven't covered yet—the way you think, move and relax.

I've been told that even when I was a child it was clear that I had an intuitive ability to help people with their health and wellness. I was always coming up with tips and bossing around my family, friends and even strangers to try to make them healthier. What I saw even then, and what I see so often in patients now, is that how you live your life can lead to accelerated aging and disease—or counteract it. In balance, our thoughts and emotions, the energy we expend exercising and the energy we save resting can all affect how well—or badly—we age. Absolutely the final piece of the puzzle in reversing the signs of aging therefore is to live an anti-aging lifestyle.

As such, this last section isn't so much a step-by-step plan, but rather advice you should live by day in, day out to help keep your body looking, feeling and acting younger and your mind feeling calm, relaxed and happy. Do that and you won't just reverse the signs of aging—you'll also have mastered the art of aging well.

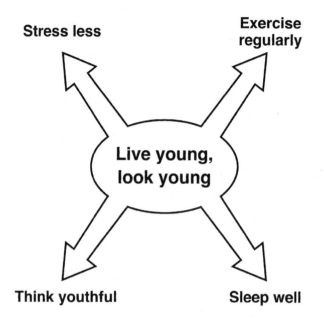

THE STRESS AND AGING CONNECTION

When I think about premature aging, what comes to mind after seeing thousands of patients is that our biggest enemy is stress. It's something we are faced with every day, but there is good stress and bad stress. Good stress keeps us going and motivates us, even improves our performance; but bad stress, the type that goes on and on, and over which you feel you have no control, drags us down, causing great harm to our health, wellness and the rate at which we age. During this type of stress, our very delicate adrenal glands set off a chemical cascade that has both physical and mental effects—and that, left to get out of control, ages your body in many ways.

Stress can make the skin look and act older

Cortisol produced during stress thins the skin; it also weakens the skin's barrier, making it sensitive, prone to irritation, at a higher risk of rosacea and also more likely to become dehydrated—ironically, though, oil production can also increase during stress, increasing the risk of adult acne. Stress also narrows blood vessels so the skin looks paler and more sallow, and, because the body diverts energy to more essential tasks, cell turnover slows down, making the skin look dull. Plus, stress creates frown lines. Chronic frowning, which you will naturally do when you're worried about something, folds the skin in ways that can cause deep permanent lines over time.

Stress affects the gut

Not only can it wreak havoc with bowel function, stress can directly impact the gut bacteria—decreasing levels of healthy forms, such as *Bacteroides* and *Lactobacillus*, and increasing levels of bugs that cause gut-flammation. Stress can also damage the gut lining and is therefore implicated in the development of leaky gut (see page 26).

Stress increases inflammation

There are many ways this happens, but notably stress causes changes deep down in the immune system that means it actually produces more pro-inflammatory cells when we're stressed.[1] Genes that trigger inflammation also become more active.

Stress unbalances hormones

Cortisol rises at stressful times, but when cortisol is high, insulin remains low, so you have sugar in the bloodstream in case you need to run away or fight an attack. But, don't forget, sugar directly ages the skin via glycation (where glucose binds to collagen fibers) and the production of AGEs (see page 72). Stress also creates an imbalance between estrogen and progesterone that can negatively affect the skin. And, don't forget its devastating effect on the adrenal glands that control so much of our hormone function.

Stress directly ages the cells

Remember those telomeres I mentioned back in Chapter 3? They are the ones that determine fundamentally how fast you age, and stress damages them. The higher your levels of cortisol, the shorter your telomeres. Interestingly, research has shown that those who worry about stress and what might happen have an even higher rate of telomere damage than those who are stressed but don't worry about it,[2] which brings me nicely to my next point.

MANAGING STRESS

The key to fighting stress is not just eliminating it from your life, but learning how to manage it, not least because it can't always be eliminated. The causes of stress are often completely out of our control, such as an irate boss, a late train on the day of an important meeting or what's going on with the economy—but what is within your control is how you react to stressful situations and the subsequent response this triggers in your body. Alter your responses to stress and you can reduce the aging impact it can have on your system. Here are five things I'd suggest you try:

1) Nourish your body

You may want to turn to crutches such as sugar, alcohol, cigarettes and caffeine when the pressure is on, but they simply stress your body further by putting pressure on the adrenal glands. Instead, fuel your body by eating balanced meals regularly (skipping meals encourages your body to release even more cortisol) and keeping stimulants to a minimum. Eat slowly—remember: eating quickly prevents proper digestion, reducing the nutrients that will enter your system. Don't give up grains. This is one thing that often surprises people—they expect me to advise them to give up all carbohydrates, but while I believe that gluten-based grains and sugary, high GI, highly refined forms of carbohydrates should play no role in your diet, gluten-free whole grains contain high levels of B vitamins that the body needs to feel calm but that get depleted when you're stressed. All of the B vitamins are vital for stress:

- **B1:** Thiamine is good for supporting blood sugar and can help to alleviate anxiety.
- **B3:** Niacin helps your feel-good hormone serotonin to increase as your body needs it.
- **B5:** Pantothenic acid helps support the adrenal glands in times of stress.
- **B12 and folic acid:** Both are important for people who have long-term anxiety, leading to depressive-like symptoms. Low levels of both have been linked to low mood and/or depression.

Whole grains and dark green leafy vegetables are also excellent sources of magnesium, another essential nutrient to fight stress. If I had to name my favorite nutrient, it would be magnesium. If magnesium were a man, I would marry him—and we'd never ever divorce as I'd be so chilled out and happy, every day would be easy like Sunday morning! Why is magnesium so magnificent? It's fundamental for a healthy body and essential for a calm one. It helps relax the body physically while reducing anxiety mentally. If you are stressed, magnesium will come to your rescue. Load your diet with sources of magnesium, or think about taking a supplement. You need 200–1,000 mg a day (if you get a tummy upset, lower your dose). It's best taken at bedtime as it can help you sleep. You can also absorb magnesium through the skin via bath salts—a super-relaxing way to boost levels. I like those from Organic Origins Spa (organicoriginsspa.com), especially their Mediterranean Sea Salt, Dead Sea Salt, Himalayan ancient sea salt and French organic sea salt, which are all rich with my love, magnesium.

2) Try the stress-supporting supplements

Magnesium is one of these; other ones that I've already mentioned include Relora (see page 137) and fish oil (see page 102), but there are a few more that I like:

- **Rhodiola:** This is an adaptogenic herb, which means it does what your body needs—if you need energy it will energize you; if you need calming, it will do that. It's very good at fighting stress because it calms the nerves without lowering energy or making you feel sluggish or drowsy. My patients who love it say it's perfect for that "fizzy stress" feeling—when everything is just overwhelming you and you can't think straight. Taking rhodiola just seems to take the edge off and help you regain the clarity of thought you need to get things done. Take 200 mg once or twice a day, before breakfast and lunch, when you're under pressure. You can increase to 600 mg if you're really burning the candle at both ends.

- **Ashwagandha:** Another adaptogenic herb, this is particularly good at helping with worrisome stress and it's very calming— in fact, in trials it's been shown to be as effective as some common anti-anxiety medications in its ability to create calm.[3] It also directly lowers cortisol. Take 600–1,000 mg daily when you're having symptoms. I quite often combine rhodiola with ashwagandha and another herb, Asian (or Panax) ginseng, of which the dose is 100–200 mg of standardized extract and the packaging states it contains 20–40 mg of ginecoside.

- **Phosphatidylserine:** When you're about to go through a period of stress—you know it's coming, you can't avoid it, but you'd like to reduce some of the damage it can have on your body—this is the supplement to choose. It's a cortisol blocker, limiting the amount that you produce as a reaction to pressure. Remember, cortisol is the Goldilocks hormone: you need just the right amount in your body; too little and you'll be drained, too much and you'll be frazzled—phosphatidylserine helps regulate things so neither occurs. Take 400 mg a day.

3) Don't catastrophize

Two women are stuck in traffic, one is freaking out and worried that she'll never move. In her head, she is envisioning that being late will lead to her being fired. Next she imagines how she won't get another job and will lose her home … The other person puts on the radio and sings along, figuring if the traffic doesn't start moving in 10 minutes, she'll call the office and let them know there's a problem. Same situation, two completely different reactions—the first more aging than the last. This type of thinking is called catastrophizing and it's very common—but a technique called mindfulness can help stop it.

Mindfulness helps you find a stillness in yourself. It sees you bringing yourself into the present, so you're not fretting about the past or worrying about the future. Either use it when stress strikes, or do a daily mindfulness exercise, which helps actually change your mindset so you are more likely to focus your thoughts more into the present and not go off into a spiral of worry. Try the exercises below:

- **The five senses:** Wherever you are, spend a minute thinking about each of the following in turn: what you can see, what you can hear, what you can smell, what you can feel and what, if anything, you can taste. Don't judge the responses to any of those questions, just feel each of the things.
- **Body scanning:** Lie down with your eyes closed. Slowly scan up and down your body for tightness and soreness. If you find a tight spot, stop and breathe into it until it relaxes. You might also imagine healing white light radiating into the spot.
- **Object meditation:** Choose an object—it could be something on your desk, something natural like a pebble, even a piece of food (many people use a raisin to do this exercise). Spend several minutes observing every aspect of it: shape, hues, textures, smells, taste (if relevant). Use all your senses. Focus on intricate detail.

4) Meditate

Meditation has been practiced in Eastern cultures for centuries, and it's an amazing way to control, strengthen and relax the mind. It's also extremely beneficial for fighting aging and has actually been shown to increase the length of the telomeres (see page 86). In a study at UCLA, for example, a type of meditation called Kirtan Kriya (pronounced keer-tun kree-a) was shown to reduce stress and improve mental well-being of those who tried it, as well as increase levels of a substance called telomerase by 43 percent—that was almost 40 percent more than people who merely relaxed by listening to music.[4] Telomerase is the enzyme that repairs the telomeres; the higher your level, the more resistant to aging you are likely to be.

I particularly like to meditate myself young with Kirtan Kriya because it's very quick to do—just 12 minutes a day practicing is enough to produce that anti-aging response. It's also a type of active meditation that's easy for anyone to master—even if, like so many of my patients, you're a workaholic who finds it very hard to switch off. Here's what you need to do:

- Sit comfortably with your spine straight and your arms placed out in front of you, palms toward the ceiling. You can literally do this meditation anywhere you feel comfortable, but you do need to speak out loud, so I wouldn't recommend doing it on the bus or train! Repeat the following sounds out loud for two minutes in your normal voice: Saa ... Taa ... Naa ... Maa ...

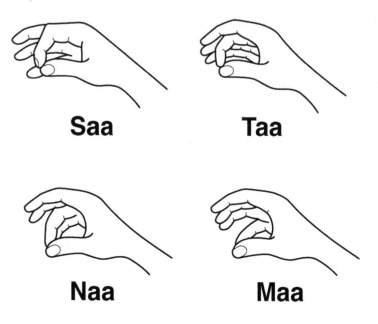

Saa   **Taa**

Naa   **Maa**

- As you make each sound, touch your fingers in turn with the tip of your thumb:
    - » On Saa—touch the first/index finger
    - » On Taa—touch the second/middle finger
    - » On Naa—touch the third/ring finger
    - » On Maa—touch your last/little finger
- When the first two minutes are over, repeat the same process but as follows:
    - » For the next two minutes repeat the words in a whisper
    - » For the next four minutes say them silently to yourself
    - » For the next two minutes whisper them
    - » For the final two minutes say them in your normal voice
- To finish, inhale deeply as you stretch your arms over your head and shake your hands, then bring them down in a sweeping motion as you exhale.

5) Get a pet

Pets are amazing stress relievers and give you unconditional love. When I am around my dog, Mimi, who is a lovely Yorkshire terrier, I feel calmer and laugh more often. In fact, research shows that when you are with your pet, the same hormone—oxytocin—that is released when a mother looks at her baby spikes. Just three minutes of stroking their dog caused a fall in cortisol levels in pet owners.[5] Of course not everyone has the lifestyle that allows them to own a pet, but that doesn't mean you can't also benefit from a little animal therapy. Schemes like Borrow My Doggy (see www.borrowmydoggy.com) allow you to walk the pets of those who can't always do so personally, and many animal charities also need volunteer walkers or carers.

SLEEPING BEAUTY

Lack of sleep is something that affects almost everyone at some point. It can be related to stress, mind chatter, hormonal fluctuations—and, very often, is caused by worrying that you can't sleep! But the less you sleep, the faster you age.

There is a reason why it's called beauty sleep. Nighttime is when skin is abuzz with surges of human growth hormone and other substances that lead to the formation of collagen and the repair of some of the DNA damage that occurs every day through exposure to UV rays. The skin is also more porous at this time, meaning that any skincare on the face or body is likely to be more effective at getting to the lower levels of skin where it's actually needed. Studies have shown that poor sleepers generally have greater signs of skin aging, including more fine lines, increased pigmentation and reduced elasticity. Their skin also recovered less effectively from sun damage.[6] The signs of sleep deprivation that occur after a few days' sleep are also extremely aging. When researchers asked respondents to look at the faces of people deprived of sleep for 31 hours and describe how they looked, they said their skin was paler, they had more fine lines and wrinkles and the corners of their mouths and eyelids were drooping.[7] Of course, learning how to sleep well will reverse these signs quickly, immediately making you look younger.

Adequate sleep also reduces inflammation. It's been shown that immune cells called monocytes that make inflammatory chemicals increase their activity when we're sleep deprived.[8]

Exactly how much sleep you need to thrive is personal, but what studies show is that a healthy amount of sleep is between six and nine hours a night, with seven to eight being the amount linked to optimum health benefits. If you're not achieving that most nights, you will be aging faster than you should and you should take some steps to help support your body's sleep-promoting systems. It's the peak age-reversing time of the day, so you really want to try to make sleeping well a priority. As I tell my patients, your body wants to sleep—you just have to help it happen.

One of the most important things you can do to promote sleep is to enhance production of the hormone melatonin. This is the hormone our body produces to fall asleep, and, like so many of the hormones I discussed in Chapter 4, its production naturally falls as we age. Melatonin is also a powerful antioxidant and an important youth-boosting hormone, so it's important to keep its levels balanced.

Melatonin is produced by the pineal gland in the brain. Its production revs up as light falls and switches off when we are exposed to daylight. The problem is many of our modern habits interfere with this natural response—the blue light given off by devices such as smartphones and tablets, for example, switches off melatonin production. In studies it's been shown that two hours of evening use of a device that emits blue light cuts melatonin production by 22 percent[9] and in some people that can be enough to interfere with sleep. Instigating what's called an electric sundown can help re-stimulate melatonin production. This means turning off all gadgets at a set time—normally around two hours before the time you want to fall asleep.

Do a light audit in your bedroom. The effect of your electric sundown will be counteracted if your bedroom is exposed to light. Go in there at your normal bedtime and turn the lights off. Give it a minute or two for your eyes to adjust, then see how much you can see. If you can see across the room when the lights are off, or, even worse, actually read a book, or you have obvious bright lights like those from a clock radio, then you need to darken your room to trigger optimum melatonin release. Try darker curtains or an eye mask and remove any electronic light sources.

In the US, you can also buy melatonin supplements, which you can use to regulate sleep for short periods. Take 1–3 mg one hour before you want to sleep. Melatonin is not sold in the UK but it can be prescribed by a doctor for some sleep problems. You can also try drinking a little tart cherry juice, which contains natural melatonin levels. In studies, people consuming 8 oz (225 g) of the juice morning and night extended their sleep time by 85 minutes a night.[10] Remember, though, it must be tart cherry juice from a type of cherry called the Montmorency to get results. You can also buy this in supplement form.

Change Your Bedding

Just as I can spot what people are eating from signs on their face, I can also spot what side they sleep on. People always develop more fine lines on the side of their face that rests on the pillow. We change position regularly while we sleep and that movement causes the skin on the face to crease, eventually creating a permanent line in the skin. People who sleep on their front are always more wrinkled than those who sleep on their back. I suggest to many of my patients that they swap to silk pillowcases, which reduce the amount the skin folds and creases. Applying your antioxidant serums and a rejuvenating moisturizer before bed also helps reduce damage. Dehydrated skin will crease more and doesn't spring back as well.

Whatever you sleep on, though, change the pillowcase once a week, twice if your skin or hair are oily. Bacteria can build up on your pillowcase over time and you then spend six to eight hours a night lying on those bugs, which can be a common cause of breakouts. If you only ever get blemishes on one side of your face and if it's the side you sleep on, your pillow might be one reason why.

There are, of course, other ways to boost how well you sleep. The herb valerian root is particularly good at tackling sleep that's associated with stress and anxiety, as it helps calm the mind as well as the body. The starting dose is 400 mg taken before bed.

If you do wake up at night or have trouble nodding off, don't stress about it—one of the most common reasons that the odd sleepless night turns into insomnia is that we start to worry that we're not asleep. If those thoughts come into your head, using any of the mindfulness exercises in this chapter can help bring your mind into the present and help you fall back to sleep.

EXERCISE

If you want to age well, you need to move your body. Movement equals flow and nourishment; not moving equals blockage and stagnation, which in Traditional Chinese Medicine leads to disease. When we don't move, we don't stimulate lymphatic drainage, our circulation is poor, and our mind and body are stuck—move, though, and there isn't an aspect of aging that won't benefit.

Exercise helps fight stress, it promotes sleep, it triggers the release of human growth hormone (hGh) and lowers levels of cortisol in the body. Exercise makes the cells more responsive to insulin-lowering sugar levels in the system, reduces levels of inflammation in the body and keeps those telomeres healthy and long. In fact, people exercising for an average of 199 minutes a week had telomeres the equivalent of 10 years younger than people moving for fewer than 16 minutes a week.[11] It also keeps the gut regular and boosts the microbiome.[12]

Most important, though, is how exercise directly affects the way the skin ages. What it does here is quite astonishing—if anything is going to convince you that exercise is a vital anti-aging tool, it's what you're about to read in this paragraph. According to studies at Canada's McMaster University, the skin of people who work out regularly actually looks completely different from that of people of the same age who don't. In their trials, the skin of exercisers in their 40s looked more like the skin of 20–30 somethings. They had a thinner stratum corneum, which indicated better cell renewal, and the dermis was thicker than that of non-exercisers.[13] Even more amazingly, when the same McMaster team asked a group of sedentary people to start exercising, they found their skin started to take on the same youthful properties—they actually turned back time on their faces. The researchers think that substances called myokines, which increase in numbers in the skin as we work out, actually instruct the cells to act younger. Add this to the fact that circulation is also raised when you work out, giving skin a youthful glow, and the fact that exercise helps promote bone growth (how fast the face ages also depends on having a healthy bone mass) and you can see why the authors of another trial at Germany's Saarland University Clinic called it "striking" how much younger exercisers looked compared to sedentary peers of the same age.[14]

This doesn't mean you need to live in the gym 24/7 though. In the McMaster trial, the new exercisers were working out just twice a week for 30 minutes at a moderate pace. As you'll see below, other studies have also shown that moderate exercise is more anti-aging than going all out, all the time. Nor do you have to start taking up running if you dread the thought. Anti-aging exercise must be something you enjoy and that leaves you feeling good after you've done it, otherwise you're likely to produce more stress hormones dreading your workout than you counteract doing it! The exercises I love include Pilates and swimming. If you enjoy running or cycling, though, then that's what's likely to be anti-aging for you. However, there are some exercises that have been shown to have some specific effects on how fast the body ages.

High-Intensity Interval Training (HIIT)

This type of workout is normally short, fast and hard, and it can combine short bursts of cardiovascular moves, such as sprinting or cycling, with short, slow recovery sessions or, if you're strength training, involve fast weight-training moves with limited rest between them. It's great to fit HIIT into the busiest of lives, but it's also the type of workout shown to cause the biggest rise in levels of hGh. HIIT workouts are also proven to improve insulin sensitivity. You shouldn't make all of your sessions HIIT type workouts, though—this can lead to overtraining, which, as you'll see shortly, can actually age the body. Do no more than two or three sessions lasting 20 minutes or less weekly.

Yoga

Yoga lowers cortisol and two 90-minute sessions a week have now been shown to also reduce levels of inflammatory markers in people's systems by 20 percent.[15] Yoga can also help aid gut health—twisting moves help rev up digestion and detoxification, while deep breathing massages the gut and helps encourage elimination.

Whole-body vibration

These vibrating platforms upon which you sit, stand or do moves, such as squats, lunges and press-ups, are often used in the elderly as they are low impact but allow for a whole-body workout. As such, their effects on aging have been extensively studied and they have been shown to improve bone density, build muscle mass and stimulate cell activity in ways that counteract the general signs of aging in the body. They also influence hormone levels, raising hGh and decreasing levels of cortisol.

Walking

Studies have shown that walking just 15 minutes a day increases lifespan by 3 years,[16] which is proof that exercise doesn't need to be intense to get results. One reason why is likely to be related to the findings of Finnish research. In trials, men who did moderate exercise, such as walking, gardening and bowling, had longer telomeres than those doing more vigorous moves, such as running or cycling.[17] Another study from the University of Maryland has shown similar results—those doing moderate amounts of exercise (burning around 1,000–3,500 calories a week) had longer telomeres than those working out to extremes or doing nothing at all.[18]

Exercise carefully

The two studies above show something important. When it comes to fighting aging, the right amount of exercise will turn back time, but do too much and you don't get the same anti-aging boost. But that's not the only anti-aging mistake to avoid. Here are seven more:

1) Working out with injuries

Any kind of injury triggers inflammation in the body—this is natural and essential to heal the body, but if you keep working out instead of letting the body heal you increase your risk of triggering the more chronic form of harmful inflammation.

2) Not resting between sessions

Exercise tones the body by damaging the muscles slightly and as they repair they strengthen and grow—the older you get, though, the longer this process takes. Doing back-to-back sessions can lead to inadequate repair, and again, trigger inflammation. That doesn't mean you shouldn't work out every day if you want to, but alternate sessions so you don't do two hard workouts back to back, and work different body parts on different days so one can be repairing while you focus on another. Also don't attempt to do more than you're fit enough to achieve—that might mean trying to run too far, lift weights that are too heavy, or even push yourself into yoga positions you haven't worked up to.

3) Not getting the right balance

Normally, exercise reduces levels of stress hormones in the body, but if you have an extremely stressful job and then head immediately to do very, very hard exercise, you can trigger the opposite response and raise stress levels further. One classic sign that this is happening is if you start to gain weight around your middle, despite your workout efforts. If this is happening, think about introducing less stressful forms of exercise such as yoga, Pilates, ballet workouts or walking into your regimen—or at the very least take time to switch off from the day before you start an intense workout.

4) Getting too thin

The more fat you have in your face, the younger you look—particularly as you get a little older. According to research published in the journal *Plastic and Reconstructive Surgery*, after the age of 40 having a very low Body Mass Index (BMI) adds years to the face.[19] Like cortisol (page 128), think like Goldilocks about weight: not too little, not too much; aim for just what's right for your body type and natural set point.

5) Not staying cool and hydrated

This actually causes the gut to become temporarily permeable as it attempts to cool you down. This triggers a mini attack of leaky gut (see page 26), which lets those larger inflammatory particles enter the system, increasing inflammation and risk of intolerance. Stay hydrated when you work out and don't overdo it in very high temperatures. Taking non-steroidal anti-inflammatory drugs, such as ibuprofen, before exercise also temporarily increases gut permeability, which is another reason why you shouldn't work out if you have an injury.

6) Exercising in make-up

When cosmetics mix with sweat they can break down and irritate the skin. On top of that, make-up and oily skincare products can stop sweat from leaving the skin effectively, which could increase your risk of breakouts. It's best to remove make-up before you work out and then apply a hyaluronic acid gel or serum afterward to replace the water lost.

7) Working out without sunscreen

If you run, cycle, walk or do any other exercise outside, it's vital that you protect your skin with a 50 SPF sunscreen. In a study of marathon runners conducted by experts at the medical University of Graz, Austria, it was found that they had more age spots and signs of sun damage than non-runners.[20] Partly this is because they were spending more time outside than other people, but sweat also increases UV absorption by the skin, making exposure during exercise potentially more harmful. Remember: UV damage causes up to 80 percent of premature aging—if you're not protecting your skin while you work out, you're counteracting many of the benefits that exercise can have on the skin.

THINK YOUTHFUL—
AND YOU WILL BE YOUTHFUL

I just want to make it clear that I don't think aging is a bad thing. With age comes wisdom, experience and enlightenment, which can be truly youthful, sexy and empowering. As we age what we should aim to achieve is a good quality of life that allows us to embrace all the things we've learned over the years. However, many of us start to think in ways that mean this doesn't happen—but we now know that the way you think, act and behave can impact on how well you age. Think young and you will look and feel younger.

The most famous experiment proving this was done by psychologist Ellen Langer in 1979. She asked a group of elderly men to live in a house like it was 1959—their heyday. Everything around them—the decoration, the technology, the music, their clothes—took them back to their prime of life. After a week the men stood straighter, walked faster, had better hearing and a higher IQ. Acting younger had literally turned back their body age.[21] This is something I'm always telling my patients: the power of the mind and its ability to make things happen is immense. If you think something, you can make it happen—if you start to think and act younger, your body will follow suit.

I'm not saying that you should be the oldest person at Burning Man or still wearing crop tops at 75 (unless that's your aim in life, in which case go for it), but many people adopt the idea that your life should change just because you've gotten older—that you should stop doing things you love, or acting in certain ways not because your body can't do it, but because it's not the thing done at your age. There's no doubt that this kind of thinking and attitude makes you age faster than you should. Be happy with who you are—who you are is a gift and the more "you" you are, the better life will be. But that's not the only way to think youthful. Here are some other ways to reprogram your old thoughts into young, positive ones:

1) Find the good in getting older

If you think you're going to age badly, you will. It's not just me saying that—research at Yale University found exactly the same thing.[22] In the trial, people who couldn't see any positives in getting older tended to die 7.5 years earlier than those who thought more about the good things to come. While they didn't explore why, other research may explain it: positive thinking extends telomeres (see page 86). It's been shown that pessimists, who tend to focus on the negatives in life, have shorter telomeres than optimists who can see the good in situations.[23]

2) Start saying yes more often

As we get older we tend to say no to more new opportunities. Not only does this see us falling into a rut of only doing things we did in the past (rather than moving with the times), it also increases the speed at which life passes us by. The brain needs novelty to thrive. Routine slowly kills off your brain cells, not to mention the fun in life. Stay young brained by trying something new every single week—it doesn't need to be anything extreme; just trying a food you've never had before or walking down a different road on the way to work and noticing what's around you is enough to create some novelty in your life.

3) Investigate and be curious

Curiosity is another trait we tend to lose as we age. We stop questioning and learning, and someone with an old brain will hear about something new and just think, "Meh, not relevant to my life," even in their 20s. Youthful thinkers want to know what it is, in case they are missing out on something fun. Life should be an adventure, big or small, and asking questions and learning new things is all a part of this. Recapturing your inquisitive nature makes you feel younger.

4) Don't tell your body it's getting old

Sighing as you sit down, grunting as you stand up as if it's a big effort, or blaming the fact that you can't find your car keys on age, rather than the fact that you were talking on the phone when you came home and threw them somewhere different, tells your body you are expecting it to underperform with age. Your brain likes to please you in life—if it thinks you're expecting your body to slow down, the brain will make that happen. Again, our proof comes from Yale: in a trial published in the journal *Psychology and Aging,* seniors reading words such as "forgetful" responded worse on memory tests than those given more positive words to read, such as "wise."[24] Tell your body it's aging well, and it will.

5) Don't do "old speak"

"I can't wear that, I can't do that, I can't go there … I'm too old." If you've caught yourself saying any of these things, enough already. We've hopefully stopped beating ourselves up if we don't have bodies that look like the supermodels—yet 66 percent of us beat ourselves up for getting older.[25] We must stop falling into traps thinking that we can't do things because we've reached a certain age. Think about this: all those stereotypes you're thinking about are based on the way people aged in the past, not the way we age now. In your great-grandparents' generation it was extremely rare for a woman in her 40s to have a baby—now it's commonplace. In our society 50- and 60-year-olds look like Meryl Streep, Sandra Bullock, Ellen DeGeneres, Helen Mirren and Madonna. Think about what you *can* do, not what you *should* do, and aim to enjoy life every single day. Don't grow old before your time because you don't have to, and remember, you are only ever as old as you think you are—so think young.

That's the external side of turning back time. Now, let's move back to the inside and the foods you can eat that help you turn back the clock; trust me, eating yourself young is a lot easier and tastier than you could ever believe.

CHAPTER 7

THE AGE-REVERSING EATING PLAN

Every time my patients get to this point of our treatment plan, they want to know how to keep up the results. My answer is to follow an age-reversing eating plan that's packed with anti-aging nutrients.

Food is your daily medicine—every fruit, vegetable, vitamin, mineral and macronutrient, such as protein, carbohydrate or fat, has a role to play in the health of the body, and the aging ability of the skin. By choosing foods with the most powerful anti-aging effects, you can help to ensure that practically every mouthful you eat is turning back time on your body clock.

A youth-boosting eating plan will clear, correct and protect you against premature fine lines, wrinkles, sagging and pigmented skin, and work alongside all the steps you've taken so far. Transform your diet and you can forget your age—age is just a number, youth is what you see on your skin. And this is how to achieve it.

The plan that follows is based upon the foods that maximize both health and beauty. It also helps walk you through the first 28 days of the Gut-Balancing CCP Plan, and supports the changes within the other plans, showing how easy and tasty it can be to give up the main dietary causes of digest-aging, such as gluten, dairy, sugar, processed foods and an excess of omega-6 fats. It's the perfect plan to base your eating on as you progress through the book.

You'll be eating three main meals a day, with a beauty burst of juicing in between to feed your cells with extra greens and other natural boosts. Every time we consume a full meal or snack too much, our digestion must work harder and harder; by constantly snacking, you can overstress digestion, which makes it sluggish. This can then potentially cause a buildup of undigested food in the digestive tract, which can then cause problems such as fermentation, bloating, toxicity buildup and a potential imbalance of bacteria that can upset everything. Juices, however, are readily digested by the body and nourish the cells within, avoiding this effect.

THE FOODS TO CHOOSE FROM

Antioxidants

Basically fruits and vegetables: eat as many as you can consume at every meal.

These should be the mainstay of your meals, taking up at least half of your plate. Also eat as many different types as you can—I personally try to include five to six different varieties at every meal. Do, however, focus mainly on vegetables. While fruit is extremely healthy, too much can raise sugar levels in your diet. Aim for at least twice as many servings of vegetables a day as fruit, if not more.

While raw vegetables are fine during the day, at night it's best to lightly steam them. Digestion starts to slow at night and steamed vegetables are easier for your system to break down. This might surprise you as it's often believed that raw vegetables are better for us, but we actually absorb higher levels of nutrients from some vegetables, such as carrots and tomatoes, after they've been cooked. I prefer steaming or steam frying to boiling. To steam fry, heat a small amount of coconut oil in the bottom of a shallow pan with a lid. Add your vegetables and sauté them until they start to sizzle. Now add a tablespoon or two of liquid such as water, coconut milk or a bone broth. Don't add too much—you're not trying to boil the food in it, just create steam. Put the lid on the pan and steam for a few minutes until your vegetables are ready to eat.

Many of the nutrients in vegetables are found in the peel, so, where possible, I suggest not peeling vegetables such as potatoes, sweet potatoes and carrots. Potato peel, for example, combines a double digest-aging–fighting combination of fiber and nutrients, such as vitamin C, magnesium, vitamin B6 and zinc, which keep your skin smooth and silky. Of course you do need to wash everything extra well if you're not eating organic to reduce exposure to any pesticides left on the skin.

When you are planning your meals for the day, aim for a good mix of the following anti-aging families:

- **Glow givers:** If you want your skin to glow, increase your intake of red, orange and yellow vegetables, such as sweet potatoes, carrots, butternut squash, red peppers and citrus fruit. Researchers at Scotland's University of St. Andrews showed that eating two extra servings daily of orange, yellow or red foods, which contain substances called carotenoids, markedly altered skin tone to create a natural healthy glow. It took just six weeks to show effects.[1]

- **Line-fighting leaves:** This means dark green leafy vegetables, such as spinach, kale and watercress: these are an excellent source of magnesium, one of my favorite minerals, and in Japanese studies women with the highest intake of green (and yellow) vegetables in their diet also had the youngest-looking skin— particularly around the eyes.[2] It's believed the fact that they help your skin create its own natural SPF is behind the effect. Watercress gets its own special mention here because when experts at William Paterson University in New Jersey ranked 41 vegetables for nutrient potential, watercress came out on top— that's right, even above kale![3]

- **Dirty hormone fixers:** These include the cruciferous vegetables, such as cabbage, cauliflower, Brussels sprouts and broccoli. Amazing detoxifiers, these help boost the health of your liver and are particularly important for balancing hormones. Other excellent detoxifiers include onions and leeks, which supply the sulfur the liver needs to process toxins out of the system.

- **Bacteria-boosting prebiotics:** These help feed the good bacteria in the gut. In addition to onions and leeks, this group includes Jerusalem artichokes, dandelion leaves, asparagus, chicory and bananas. In one study, simply adding these foods alone to people's diets raised levels of their good bacteria numbers by 133 million in a week.[4]

- **Power-packed berries:** Berries are one of the best fruits to eat as their slight natural bitterness means they have a lower GI than many fruits. Many people reach for blueberries for anti-aging, but red berries contain a magic ingredient called ellagic acid, a polyphenol that's been shown to counteract the damage UV light does to skin, triggering wrinkle formation. It actually stops the release of collagen-destroying MMP (matrix metalloproteinase) that normally occurs when UV hits the skin.[5]

Gut-friendly grains

Eat a fist-sized serving at most meals.

I've said before how surprised my patients are when I tell them that they absolutely must eat carbohydrates because whole grains are an incredible source of antioxidants. They also contain so many of the nutrients that you need to fight inflamm-aging, such as the B vitamins or magnesium. All of the following are examples of good gluten-free grains (don't forget you can also include products made from these, such as breads, noodles, cereals and wraps):

- **Amaranth:** Actually a seed, this becomes sticky when it's cooked. This doesn't make it the best alternative to foods such as pasta, but it does make it an excellent hot breakfast cereal (see page 234) or base for puddings. It's high in protein, which makes it a great building block for healthy skin, but it is still a high GI grain, so it will raise blood-sugar levels, which is something you want to try to avoid. Serving it with a little fat or extra protein, such as eggs, will counteract this.

- **Buckwheat:** Despite its name, it doesn't actually contain wheat—in fact, it's a relative of rhubarb. It has a chewy texture and a nutty taste, which goes well with meat and vegetables. It also makes a good flour for foods such as pancakes (though double-check labels as some buckwheat flours are mixed with wheat). Soba noodles are also made from buckwheat (but again double-check labels) and make a good alternative to wheat-based noodles in soups or stir-fries. Buckwheat is high in a circulation-boosting antioxidant called rutin that helps improve circulation—great for giving skin a glow.
- **Quinoa:** Technically this is a seed rather than a grain, but we'll include it here as it makes a good base for so many meals. Pronounced "keen-wa," it makes a great alternative to pasta or couscous in any dish. It also works well as a hot breakfast cereal. When you cook with quinoa, rinse it first. It's covered with a bitter compound called saponin, which not only gives it a bitter taste if it's not removed, but can also irritate the gut.
- **Rice:** Brown, wild, red, black or basmati are the more skin-friendly varieties to choose as they contain higher levels of fiber and nutrients and/or a lower GI than normal white rice.
- **Teff:** This nutrient-rich grain grown in Ethiopia makes an excellent base for breads and hot breakfast cereals. Right now it's commonly sold as flour, or you can buy a number of ready-made products that contain it, such as breads and cereals.

Don't forget that other good ways to replace gluten in meals include potatoes and other tubers, legumes and beans.

Power proteins

Eat a portion at every meal.

Protein is the building block of beauty. It's the substance from which skin, hair and nails are formed, and without adequate levels, all of these three things will suffer. All forms of protein are great for skin, but the ones that I think have skin superpowers include:

- **Bone broth:** This is an excellent source of protein and like the cell whisperer for anti-aging. It contains natural doses of collagen, which heal the gut and prevent gut-flammation, and of course build strong, wrinkle-resisting skin. It's also packed with anti-aging minerals, such as calcium and magnesium, and its chemical composition makes it very easy for your body to absorb.

- **Eggs:** I'm a big fan of eggs as they are complete nutrient powerhouses, containing a whopping eight major vitamins and a selection of minerals. They also contain lecithin that helps repair skin tissue and keep the cell membranes strong to slow down the aging process. However, they are one of the foods that comes up time and time again when I test people for intolerances. If you suspect they are a problem food for you, it's okay to swap in another protein food. Choose free-range eggs if you can; the hens eat a varied diet and the extra nutrients also pass on to you.

- **Oily fish:** Salmon, anchovies, mackerel, sardines and trout are excellent proteins and rich sources of omega-3 fats that help combat wrinkles but also fight acne, eczema and skin dryness. On top of this, of course, they are possibly the most powerful anti-inflammatory foods you can eat. They are one of the few foods that contain vitamin D, and increasing your intake of this can help prevent dark circles under the eyes.

- **Poultry:** An excellent lean choice of protein, turkey and chicken also contain a specific skin super weapon. The slightly darker meat that you find around the bone in chicken legs or thighs is a concentrated source of zinc that helps promote skin regeneration. Don't just eat the whiter breast meat if you want the whole beauty boost.

- **Beans/legumes:** These include all the different varieties of lentils you can buy and also the many different types of beans. Each of these can have a slightly different taste and texture, and you could easily go a week adding a different lentil or bean to your meals and never get bored. You'll also look younger—when

Australian researchers[6] looked at what foods were linked to younger-looking skins, legumes were one of them.

- **Red meat:** Red meat provides heme iron, the type our body finds easiest to absorb. If your iron levels are low, your skin will look paler and your thyroid can start to underperform, leading to dry, thinning skin. Low iron levels are also linked to higher levels of anxiety, and, as I've explained, stress is extremely aging to the skin.

- **Soy:** Like eggs, some people do find they react to soy, but if you don't have problems with it, it's an excellent skin boost due to its estrogen-mimicking abilities. In a study looking at what happened when women added soy to their diet, it was found they had less dryness, better skin tone and fewer wrinkles.[7] Remember, though, fermented foods, such as miso, tempeh or natto, are better than plain tofu or soy milk/yogurt, so do add a good variety of types.

Beauty oils and super seeds

These foods contain the healthy fats that your skin needs for correct hydration. We have gotten used to eating low-fat foods and are now almost scared of adding any fat, even the healthiest ones, to our meals. If, however, you increase levels of the right fats—the unsaturated fats, omega-3 oils and coconut oil—you will notice your skin looks plumper, lines and wrinkles start to fade and your skin simply takes on a healthier, more youthful look. Adding fat to a meal also helps keep you full and feeling satisfied afterward. Aim to add a small serving to most, if not all, your meals. Here are some of my favorite sources:

- **Avocado:** An excellent source of monounsaturated fats that fight inflammation, avocados also contain glutathione that soothes the gut lining and helps the liver with its daily detoxification tasks. Avocados also contain antioxidants called lutein and zeaxanthin, which have been shown to protect the skin against sun damage.[8]

- **Algaes:** It might surprise you that these contain doses of essential fats. I can't say enough good things about these green superfoods, which include chorella and spirulina. They are packed with chlorophyll that helps oxygenate the skin, but they also contain vitamin D, vitamin K, selenium, folic acid, iodine, iron and vitamin B12—all essential nutrients for the health of the skin and hormone balance.
- **Chia seeds:** These tiny omega-3–packed seeds make an excellent base for hot breakfast cereal or as an addition to smoothies. Their high content of omega-3 is not their only beauty benefit though—they also contain vitamin E, zinc and stress-busting magnesium.
- **Flaxseed and flaxseed oil:** Rich in alpha-linolenic acid, which your body converts to anti-inflammatory agents in the body, flax is one of the richest vegetable sources of omega-3 fats. Flaxseeds are great sprinkled over salads or added to smoothies—the oil makes a great base for salad dressing (don't cook with it, though, as its structure changes when heated).
- **Nuts and nut butters:** The perfect mix of skin-strengthening protein and heaps of healthy fat in tiny delicious bundles, nuts are an incredible skin food. From super-sweet cashews, which satisfy any leftover sugar cravings, to full-flavored Brazil nuts, just one or two provide all the vital skin-supporting selenium you need in one day.
- **Olives and olive oil:** These are rich in a substance called oleic acid, which boosts skin health. Olives also contain a fat called squalene, which also helps to keep skin looking plump.
- **Coconut oil:** This fat is truly a superfood. It contains a substance called lauric acid, which has been shown to be antimicrobial and boost immunity. It is one of the best oils for cooking with as its structure does not change at a high heat.

Herbs, spices and seasonings
Add to every meal.

These are so powerful at fighting aging in the body I like to add them to every meal. That's why you will find so many spice-based recipes in the plan that follows—each one of them is like taking a mini dose of natural medicine. If you don't normally like spicy foods, reduce the quantities of spices, such as chili powder, cayenne and ginger, which tend to add more heat to dishes, and focus instead on the flavorful spices, such as cumin and turmeric.

Simple ways to spice up any meal quickly are the Chili Power "salsa" (see page 256) and the Harissa Mix (see page 258), or try a serving of kimchi. Simply add these on the side, or sprinkle them over any meal. Herbs, such as parsley, mint and cilantro, also make great additions to salads, while powdered spices, such as turmeric, cumin and cayenne, blend into scrambled eggs, juices, soups and salad dressings deliciously. Green chilies go on everything in my house! Every herb or spice will benefit your body, but here are some particularly great anti-agers:

- **Chilies:** Hot peppers, such as green and red chilies, paprika, cayenne and jalapeño are rich in vitamins A and C, and help prevent the breakdown of collagen to maintain healthy integrity of your skin.
- **Cinnamon:** This sweet spice can be added to breakfast cereals and smoothies and is packed with tons of antioxidants. It's also extremely good at lowering blood sugar, making it an excellent food for anyone with Sugar Face (see page 71).
- **Garlic:** I'm so sad I can't eat garlic—it's such a fantastic anti-aging food and specifically contains ingredients that reduce damage to skin caused by UV rays and suppress pro-inflammatory enzymes.[9]
- **Kimchi:** Not only do you get the boost of the chilies and garlic it contains, this is a fermented food, which means it's amazing

for gut health and fights digest-aging. It's also loaded with collagen-boosting vitamins A, C and E.

- **Parsley:** Rich in flavonoids called apigenins, which are shown to be anti-inflammatory and to act as free radical scavengers, parsley also contains chlorophyll that helps oxygenate the body. It's great for keeping the skin youthful.

- **Salt:** Salt is a great addition to your meals to give you flavor and especially for those who have blood pressure on the lower side as it adds a dose of minerals—I particularly like Himalayan salt or sea salts. However, still limit your consumption if you have high blood pressure.

- **Turmeric:** Absolutely my favorite beauty-boosting spice, turmeric's anti-inflammatory powers are second to none, turning back time on the skin. I add it to eggs, soups, smoothies, stews and curries.

FOUR WEEKS TO EAT YOURSELF YOUNG

The plan that follows gives you 28 days' worth of suggestions of beauty-boosting meals and snacks. I guarantee you'll be glowing with health, vitality and youth by the end of it. For all four weeks, start every day with a cup of warm water and squeeze in half a grapefruit or lemon to kickstart digestion. A dash of cinnamon or turmeric adds an extra boost.

Week 1

Day 1

- **Breakfast:** Poached, scrambled or boiled eggs with toasted teff bread, rice crackers or rice cakes. Add grilled tomatoes and red, yellow or green peppers. A beauty boost of avocado also helps keep free radicals from attacking the skin.

- **Lunch:** Chicken breast or quinoa with a serving of Perfect Skin Dip (see page 256) and crudités of beauty boosters rich in vitamin C, such as green pepper, red pepper and carrots.
- **Afternoon snack:** Green Juice (repeat this daily—see recipe ideas on page 259)
- **Dinner:** Stir-fry of kale, mixed peppers, onion, mushrooms and red chili (in olive or coconut oil) topped with prawns or cashews. Serve with rice or quinoa.

Day 2
- **Breakfast:** Chia Porridge (see page 234). Such a simple recipe but with chia, nuts, berries and cinnamon, it's a skin super bowl.
- **Lunch:** Spicy Soup (see page 238). Add green chilies for a super-spice boost.
- **Dinner:** Grilled salmon fillet with a side of brown rice or quinoa, spinach, chopped tomato, onion, broccoli and mushrooms. If you're vegetarian, try a Veggie Bowl (see page 242). Pimp out both with a serving of Chili Power (see page 256) or Super Skin Mix (see page 257).

Day 3
- **Breakfast:** Teff toast with nut butter, unsweetened or homemade (see page 255). Add a mix of different berries for a sweet but low GI boost.
- **Lunch:** Salad of cubed sweet potato, pomegranate seeds, asparagus and red pepper on a bed of baby spinach. Serve with poached salmon dusted with paprika (paprika is rich in betacarotene, which gets converted to skin-boosting vitamin A). Top with pumpkin seeds for extra skin healing (if you're a vegetarian, omit the fish and add more seeds). For any salads, also add a serving of Skin-Boosting Salad Dressing (see page 257).
- **Dinner:** Mixed seafood (such as prawns, mussels, squid) or tempeh stir-fried with red pepper, sugar snap peas, zucchini, asparagus, ginger and chilies, served with wild rice or quinoa.

Day 4

- **Breakfast:** Quinoa and poached eggs topped with a beauty oil boost of smoked salmon or nuts. Add chopped red onions, broccoli and spinach to the eggs.
- **Lunch:** Green Juice (see page 259 or buy a green vegetable juice from a juice bar) with a sandwich of teff bread and sardines/tuna and sliced tomato or Nut Butter (see page 255) with banana.
- **Dinner:** Grilled fillet of any white fish or roasted red pepper topped with Lima Bean Hummus (see page 244). Add collagen-boosting roasted sweet or purple potatoes with the skins on, and spinach and asparagus.

Day 5

- **Breakfast:** Any Power Porridge (see page 234) with fresh or dried apricots and berries. Up your healthy fats in an instant by adding flaxseed or coconut oil from the suggested Superfood Power Ups (see page 235).
- **Lunch:** Hot or cooled soba noodles topped with flaked mackerel or adzuki beans and diced cucumber, spring onion and avocado. Peppery watercress makes a great garnish—and adds extra antioxidants.
- **Dinner:** Spiced Lentils (see page 244) with chicken or a serving of rice, with kale, red pepper, zucchini and sugar snap peas.

Day 6

- **Breakfast:** Omelet with a beauty boost of finely chopped red, green or yellow peppers, and lycopene-rich tomatoes. Add finely chopped green chilies, red onion and spinach for your ultimate skin saver. Serve with teff toast or a fresh arugula salad.
- **Lunch:** Salad of watercress, finely chopped kale, olives, cherry tomatoes, mint, red onion and chickpeas. Add chicken or a serving of quinoa. Remember, protein at lunch helps keep you satisfied for longer. Top with Mustard Dressing (see page 258).
- **Dinner:** Healthy Curry (see page 245) with wild rice or quinoa.

Day 7

- **Breakfast:** Scrambled eggs with Sweet Potato Cakes (see page 235), grilled tomatoes and avocado (combining tomatoes and fat boosts absorption of the youth-boosting lycopene they contain).
- **Lunch:** Chicken or Minted Quinoa (see page 239) with Lima Bean Hummus (see page 244), and "eat the rainbow" crudites of red pepper, green pepper and carrot.
- **Dinner:** Soba noodles topped with a mix of stir-fried kale, chopped tomato, onion, and grilled fish or tofu/tempeh. Serve with a little Chili Power (see page 256) on the side to spice up your antioxidants.

Week 2

Day 1

- **Breakfast:** Chia Porridge (see page 234). Add fruit if you want to.
- **Lunch:** Sandwich of buckwheat bread spread with mustard and filled with avocado or roast beef, spinach and tomato. Handful of olives or nuts to give a dose of appetite-sustaining healthy fat.
- **Dinner:** Risotto (made as per instructions on the rice packet) with sun-dried tomatoes, asparagus, mushroom and peas. Serve with grilled chicken or sprinkle with pine nuts.

Day 2

- **Breakfast:** Buckwheat Bircher (see page 236).
- **Lunch:** Nicoise-style salad with tomato, green beans, red onion, olives, tuna and/or egg, and red or sweet potatoes. Add extra avocado for a dose of beauty-boosting fat.
- **Dinner:** Butternut Squash Soup (see page 246) with a huge rainbow-based salad. For an added boost of beauty oil, sprinkle some pumpkin seeds or pine nuts on top of the soup or salad.

Day 3

- **Breakfast:** Smooth Skin Smoothie (see page 236) with rice cakes and Nut Butter (see page 255). Proof that a beauty-boosting breakfast can be made in minutes.
- **Lunch:** Salmon or a mix of lentils and seeds, served with a mixed salad of red peppers, grated carrot, watercress and baby tomatoes. Don't forget to add the Skin-Boosting Salad Dressing (see page 257).
- **Dinner:** Grilled lamb or poached eggs with mashed sweet potato (keep the skins on even if you are mashing) and a medley of hormone-balancing vegetables, such as steamed green beans, carrots, zucchini, cauliflower and broccoli.

Day 4

- **Breakfast:** Skin-food fruit salad made from any piece of fruit, chopped, a mix of berries and one tablespoon of chia seeds. Get your beauty oil boost from coconut milk or coconut yogurt and a handful of nuts or a tablespoon of Nut Butter (see page 255).
- **Lunch:** Minted Quinoa (see page 239) served with tuna or salmon (canned or fresh). Serve on a bed of line-fighting dark green leaves, such as spinach, watercress or kale—or all three.
- **Dinner:** Any white fish, grilled. Serve with black beans, a salsa of chopped tomato, onion and chili and a mix of kale, broccoli and zucchini. Vegetarians: omit the fish and serve with rice or buckwheat.

Day 5

- **Breakfast:** Scrambled eggs with quinoa and avocado. Add finely chopped tomatoes, cilantro and chopped fresh chilies for your beauty boost.
- **Lunch:** Flaked salmon or hummus served on a bed of lentils, artichokes (another great detoxifying food) and watercress, with a selection of steamed vegetables.

- **Dinner:** Mexican Peppers (see page 247) served on wild or brown rice with broccoli, kale and sugar snap peas.

Day 6
- **Breakfast:** Poached egg and spinach, avocado and grilled tomatoes, with rice crackers or teff toast.
- **Lunch:** Watercress topped with chickpeas, avocado, finely chopped parsley and red onions. Serve with fresh sardines or anchovies, or a slice of buckwheat bread.
- **Dinner:** Any fish, grilled, and served with Chickpeas with Spinach (see page 248), with added broccoli, asparagus and red pepper. Stir-fry these in coconut oil for an amazing taste boost that also hydrates your skin. If vegetarian, omit the fish and serve with quinoa, brown or wild rice, or buckwheat.

Day 7
- **Breakfast:** Any Power Porridge (see page 234). Perhaps try a dab of spirulina and sliced banana to turn your breakfast into a lean, green, age-fighting machine.
- **Lunch:** Sexy Skin Salad (see page 240). This contains pomegranate seeds—another amazing source of antioxidants shown to protect skin against sun damage.
- **Dinner:** Grilled steak or lamb with quinoa or lentils and a side of kale, cauliflower, carrots, red pepper and Brussels sprouts, stir-fried in ginger and coconut oil. Or Veggie Bowl (see page 242).

Week 3

Day 1
- **Breakfast:** Smooth Skin Smoothie (see page 236) with boiled egg and rice cakes. Dairy-free protein powders such as rice, hemp or pea are a great way to quickly protein pimp any smoothie.
- **Lunch:** Brown or wild rice (warm or cooled) with avocado, sun-dried tomato, spring onion and prawns, or a mix of sunflower seeds and nuts.

- **Dinner:** Butternut Squash Soup (see page 246) or Spicy Soup (see page 238) with a large green salad. A sprinkle of turmeric added just before serving adds even more of an age-fighting boost.

Day 2

- **Breakfast:** Teff toast, rice crackers or rice cakes with sliced boiled egg. Any piece of fruit or some berries, or for a zingy start to the day, add a serving of Super Skin Mix (see page 257) or Chili Power (see page 256).
- **Lunch:** Sexy Skin Salad (see page 240). It's so good, you eat it twice!
- **Dinner:** Veggie Bowl (see page 242) or quinoa topped with olives, flaked salmon, broccoli, artichoke, tomato and asparagus.

Day 3

- **Breakfast:** Apple or banana with nut butter. Power Porridge (see page 234). Today try a boost of cacao powder—it's the raw ingredient in chocolate and packed with antioxidants, but the powder has no sugar.
- **Lunch:** Butternut Squash Soup (see page 246) with chicken or boiled egg, green olives and rice crackers.
- **Dinner:** Grilled steak with lentils or Stuffed Peppers (see page 249), with a mix of leeks, zucchinis, Brussels sprouts, carrots and kale.

Day 4

- **Breakfast:** Buckwheat Bircher (see page 236).
- **Lunch:** Chicken or poached/boiled egg served with sliced tomatoes, beets and watercress. Add teff bread/rice crackers with a little Perfect Skin Dip (see page 256).
- **Dinner:** Poached or grilled salmon, or grilled mushrooms, topped with pine nuts. Top with a Super Skin Mix (see page 257) and serve with new potatoes, broccoli, zucchini, carrots, mushrooms and kale.

Day 5

- **Breakfast:** Sweet Potato Cakes (see page 235) with poached egg, served with sautéed spinach, grilled tomatoes and avocado with a pinch of Harissa Mix (see page 258).
- **Lunch:** Greek-style salad of cucumber, tomatoes, spinach and olives, topped with edamame beans and red onions. Add a beauty-boosting choice of fish (cod, tuna, halibut, sole or mackerel) for extra protein. Serve with a slice of teff bread spread with a thin layer of coconut oil. Coconut oil has amazing anti-aging and immune-boosting properties.
- **Dinner:** Spiced Noodle Soup (see page 250) with a green salad packed with line-fighting leaves (see page 206).

Day 6

- **Breakfast:** Turmeric Eggs (see page 237) with teff toast. This recipe is such an easy way to add a dose of spice to your day. Add some beets, tomatoes and spinach.
- **Lunch:** Kale and Apple Salad (see page 240). Mixing fruits into salads is a great way to deliver their antioxidants without the sudden rise of sugar that can come from eating them alone.
- **Dinner:** Garlic prawns, scallops or tofu/tempeh served with brown rice/quinoa, spinach, kale, onion, peppers and cauliflower, garnished with freshly chopped parsley.

Day 7

- **Breakfast:** A mix of berries, nuts and one tablespoon of chia seeds, mixed with a little coconut milk or coconut yogurt.
- **Lunch:** Roast beef (or other meat) or Stuffed Peppers (see page 249) with a selection of vegetables and roast potatoes; again, keep the skins for an antioxidant injection.
- **Dinner:** Cod Provençale (see page 251) served with brown rice and a medley of beauty-boosting colorful vegetables of your choice. Or try a Veggie Bowl (see page 242).

Week 4

Day 1

- **Breakfast:** Any Power Porridge (see page 234).
- **Lunch:** Minted Quinoa (see page 239) with salmon or chickpeas and watercress.
- **Dinner:** Cauliflower Pizza (see page 252) served with a "rainbow"-based salad. Using cauliflower as a pizza base is another great way to add more of this detox superstar.

Day 2

- **Breakfast:** Chia Porridge (see page 234). Add a banana or sliced oranges.
- **Lunch:** Salmon with kale and Super Skin Mix (see page 257). Power up with some Harissa Mix (see page 258) served on a bed of wild rice.
- **Dinner:** Grilled chicken or omelet with red peppers served with mashed or puréed Jerusalem artichokes (food for you and your good gut bugs), and a mix of kale, zucchini, grilled tomato and broccoli.

Day 3

- **Breakfast:** Boiled, poached or scrambled egg, asparagus, grilled tomato, avocado, and rice cakes or crackers.
- **Lunch:** Portion of brown rice or quinoa sushi with miso soup—add some strips of dried seaweed. You'll find this in most supermarkets and it gives a jolt of iodine. Serve with spirals of cucumber and chopped apple.
- **Dinner:** Chicken or tempeh with mushroom and red pepper made into kebabs, grilled and served with a side of wild rice or quinoa, broccoli and kimchi for a fermented food Power Up.

Day 4

- **Breakfast:** Nut Butter (see page 255) on teff toast, rice crackers or rice cakes. Add a side bowl of berries with chopped bananas (bananas are a prebiotic treat for your gut bacteria).
- **Lunch:** Curried Brussels Sprouts Salad (see page 241) with shredded chicken or some lima beans and seeds.
- **Dinner:** Any oily fish, grilled, or poached eggs, served with new potatoes, cauliflower and broccoli. Add some Super Skin Mix (see page 257) or Chili Power (see page 256).

Day 5

- **Breakfast:** Any Power Porridge (see page 234). Today, try boosting things with a little lucuma powder. This superfood powder from a Peruvian fruit tastes just like butterscotch.
- **Lunch:** Green Juice (see page 259) or Smooth Skin Smoothie (see page 236). Teff toast or rice crackers with mashed avocado and smoked salmon or boiled egg.
- **Dinner:** Chili and Cauliflower Rice (see page 254). Swapping normal rice for cauliflower rice is another brilliant way to add a hormonal detoxification boost to your meals.

Day 6

- **Breakfast:** Buckwheat Bircher (see page 236). Try a spoonful of coconut yogurt or Nut Butter (see page 255) to get an extra burst of beauty oil benefits.
- **Lunch:** Salad of black beans, avocado and arugula, served with salsa or a serving of Chili Power (see page 256). Add chicken or some cashews.
- **Dinner:** Roast lamb or Spiced Lentils (see page 244) served with cabbage or sauerkraut (available in many supermarkets), broccoli, Brussels sprouts, peas and sweet potato.

Day 7

- **Breakfast:** Omelet with finely chopped peppers, tomatoes and red onion with dusted paprika. Sliced sautéed skin-on potatoes or Sweet Potato Cakes (see page 235).
- **Lunch:** Salad of spinach, watercress, grated carrot and beet with avocado. Add poached salmon, tuna or Lima Bean Hummus (see page 244).
- **Dinner:** Grilled chicken or tofu with lentils. Add leeks, red pepper, asparagus, cauliflower and broccoli.

HOW TO CREATE YOUR OWN MEALS

The eating plan naturally supports all of the dietary advice within the individual CCP plans, but I'm guessing you're not going to want to follow a set diet plan for three to four months. Even if you do, I'm pretty sure that there will be an ingredient or recipe I suggest that you don't like, or a meal that just simply doesn't fit into your day. That's okay—it's very easy to adapt the plan or even create your own meals using a simple blueprint. Try to follow the tips below when you branch out on your own:

- **Antioxidants:** At every meal aim to eat 8–10 different types daily, mixing up the different anti-aging "families" (see page 205).
- **Gut-friendly grains:** Ideally at every meal, or twice daily if you'd prefer to base a meal around a starchy protein such as beans or lentils. Eat a fist-sized portion.
- **Power proteins:** Aim to eat a piece of protein, about the size of a pack of cards, at every meal.
- **Beauty oils or superseeds:** Eat two to three servings a day—for oils, it's a thimbleful, for seeds or nuts, try a small palmful.
- **Herbs and spices:** Ideally, add to every meal.

FIVE QUICK BREAKFASTS

Breakfast is called this simply because you're breaking the fast after a restorative sleep. It's the most important meal of the day for anti-aging as it helps balance stress hormones, such as cortisol, and it's also an excellent time to boost your intake of anti-aging foods. You must not skip it. However, it can take a little bit longer to make breakfasts when you're not reaching for bread or cereal—and I'm aware that mornings are often the most time-crunched part of the day. If you really are stuck for time, these breakfasts take no more than five minutes to put together and can be substituted for any other suggestion on the plan:

1. Teff or buckwheat bread with Nut Butter (see page 255) and berries.
2. Fruit and nuts with a little coconut yogurt and rice crackers.
3. Smooth Skin Smoothie (see page 236) and nuts, or Nut Butter (see page 255) and rice cakes.
4. Buckwheat Bircher (see page 236) (as it's made the night before).
5. Teff toast or rice cakes with avocado and smoked salmon.

LUNCHES

We so commonly fall into the trap of reaching for a sandwich and a bag of chips when lunchtime comes around—or we'll grab a salad with not much in it—but both of these can lead to energy dips that trigger dreadful mid-afternoon sugar cravings. Even worse is skipping lunch altogether and then reaching for that chocolate bar mid-afternoon instead of a meal. Protein is particularly essential at lunch because it helps insulin work more effectively and balances blood sugar. Adding a little fat is also a good idea.

Ideally, make your lunch at home and take it with you. As well as saving money, you'll know exactly what you are eating, and I don't just mean the food-based ingredients when I say this. Pre-packed lunches rely heavily on processed foods, which can come in packaging that contains chemicals such as BPA (see page 130). I know making your own lunch takes a little bit of time, but it's time you're investing in your health.

If it's really not possible to take lunch into work, here are four anti-aging lunches you can buy at many grocery stores:

- Portion of brown rice and fish sushi, with sliced cucumber, some sea vegetables or a low GI fruit such as an apple or some berries. Miso soup. You can also find quinoa-based sushi in Whole Foods if you have one near you.
- Fresh vegetable-based juice from a juice bar, or a fresh vegetable soup, accompanied by a portion of nuts, hummus or a boiled egg and some rice cakes.
- Any dressing-free salad with protein, such as chicken, egg or tuna, and vegetables, and a serving of quinoa, lentils or beans, etc. This type of salad is available from the self-service section of a health food store like Whole Foods.
- Baked potato with plain tuna, chicken, egg or beef chili with kidney beans. Add a salad or some fruit.

A Note About Servings

Most of the recipes in the plan serve four. If that's more food than you need, don't worry—unless otherwise stated they can be frozen or they will keep in the fridge for a day or two. It's also completely okay to repeat a meal on the plan or use leftovers for lunch the next day—do whatever works best for you. However, "batch cooking," where you prepare a few servings of a meal in one go, is one of the best ways to making cooking from scratch easy to build into your life. I always cook more than I need for a meal so I have some ready for those lazy days.

EATING OUT

If you're eating out, it can be hard to be absolutely sure what's gone into meals, especially in meals that contain sauces. Most restaurants do now pinpoint gluten-free and dairy-free meals on the menu, or the waiter can find out for you. The following meals will normally fit the bill:

- Plain grilled fish, chicken, steak or lamb with rice or potatoes and vegetables.
- Rogan josh, jalfrezi or dahl-based curries with boiled rice (wild if they offer it, or quinoa if it's on the menu), spinach and cauliflower.
- Chicken, prawns or beef stir-fried with boiled rice or rice/soba noodles.
- Sushi, sashimi, rice, soba noodles, miso soup and any seaweed-based salads.

WHAT ABOUT SNACKS?

Not surprisingly, the fat and sugar-based combinations of snacks, such as chocolate bars, chips, cakes and cookies, mean they are not on the plan. Many of us reach for these for a quick energy boost mid-afternoon, not realizing that the boost they give causes a second crash at about 6 p.m.—if you're always starving when you get home from work, or end up exhausted on the sofa every night, don't necessarily blame your workload; it might be your sugary afternoon snack that's sapping your energy.

That doesn't mean you should never snack. On the contrary, if you have lunch at noon and then don't get to eat your evening meal until 8 p.m., it's good to have a something to eat mid-afternoon. Leaving too long between meals actually triggers your body to release cortisol—yes, that's right, skipping meals is also aging!

I'm a big fan of vegetable juices mid-afternoon to give a sugar-free energy boost. I've given some recipes on page 259 to get you started, but you'll also find more in the book *Plenish: Juices to Boost, Cleanse and Heal* by Kara Rosen. If you can't juice, try having a small handful of nuts, perhaps with a piece of fruit or a little dried fruit. Vegetable-based snacks, such as kale chips, are also a good option. Or try having a little nut butter spread on an apple or banana, or hummus with crudités.

How Much Should You Eat?

As this is not a weight-loss plan, I haven't given the exact amounts of each food you should eat, but that doesn't mean you can go overboard. Meals should be satisfying but you shouldn't leave the table groaning—eating too much overburdens the digestive system and increases the risk of problems such as acid reflux and indigestion. A good rule is to follow the Japanese principle of Hara Hachi Bu, which means you put down your knife and fork when you feel about 70–80 percent full. It takes a little while for your brain to catch up, but you will soon feel fully satisfied. Always eat mindfully.

WHAT SHOULD YOU DRINK?

Where there is pollution, there needs to be dilution, so good hydration is essential to your daily routine.

In terms of drinks, water, ideally filtered, is your best choice. Water helps us flush out toxins from our bodies. Exactly how much you need varies and you can drink too much water, especially if you gulp it all at once. Instead, space it out, drinking a glass of water every two to three hours, especially if you are craving sugar. I have to make my water more interesting so I add flavor with lemon, lime, orange, sliced apple, grapefruit pieces, mint and even spices such as turmeric.

Tea is also a great skin drink as it's full of antioxidants—try green, white or black tea (use nut milks instead of dairy). Or there are so many amazing herbal teas to try. I particularly love peppermint tea as it's refreshing and invigorating—and aids digestion. Rooibos (aka red bush) is another full-flavored tea that contains antioxidants your skin will love. Chamomile helps aid sleep, while ginger is a great pep up. Another idea I love is to freeze herbal teas in ice cube trays and add these to water.

It might surprise you to hear that I don't ban coffee. It's an extremely good source of antioxidants and it's not true that it's diuretic. Don't add dairy to it though—either drink it black, use nut milks or I also particularly like coffee blended with butter or with a shot of coconut oil, which can reduce how stimulating it is. Coffee can be too intense for the adrenals in some people, so if you are extremely stressed, try chicory coffee instead—it tastes similar but is less adrenally stressful and is also an excellent source of inulin that helps gut bacteria thrive.

One thing to avoid: bottled water in plastic containers—it might seem healthy, but plastic bottles can contain the endocrine disruptor BPA (see page 130).

Know Your ORAC Values

ORAC stands for "oxygen radical absorbance capacity," which is a measurement of a food's ability to destroy the free radicals that cause damage in your body. The higher the ORAC score, the more anti-aging a food will be. Foods with extremely high scores that you should add regularly to your diet include blueberries, raspberries and blackberries. Spices have a very high ORAC values as do nuts, beans and lentils. Among the vegetables, onions, broccoli and asparagus are ORAC superstars. That's why you'll find all of these in the Age-Reversing Eating Plan.

FIVE GREAT KITCHEN GADGETS

Cooking from scratch is one of the keys to anti-aging eating. It means you can maximize nutrients and avoid additives that are often found in processed foods, but having the right equipment makes cooking from scratch much easier. Here are five gadgets that make it simple:

- **Vitamix:** This is an amazing blender allowing you to whip up smoothies, soups, nut milks and dressings in minutes. If you're going to buy a blender, this is the one I'd recommend.
- **NutriBullet:** If you don't have a lot of kitchen space, this small but powerful blender is amazing. Again, it's excellent for smoothies and soups. I've tested this directly against other blenders and for some reason the smoothies simply taste so much better!
- **A pressure cooker:** If you are short on time, pressure cookers offer the perfect solution. You can make nutrient-dense soups in just 25 fuss-free minutes.
- **A slow cooker:** If you're at work all day, the idea of cooking a meal when you get in isn't appealing. If you have a slow cooker, though, you can just put in your beauty-boosting protein, vegetables and spices and you'll arrive home to a house full of delicious smells and a goodness-packed ready-made dinner.
- **A hand blender:** A blender is a great addition to any healthy kitchen, but if you're just making small portions of things, such as salad dressings, sauces or pestos, a hand blender works better.

WHERE TO BUY

While quinoa is now in almost every supermarket, some of the foods I'm suggesting might not be so easy to buy, depending on where you live, so you may need to go to a specialty retailer or buy them online. Organic fruit and vegetables and juices can also be delivered around the country if that's easier for you. Whole Foods Market and your local farmers' markets feature an array of organic fruits and vegetables, as do national chain grocery stores.

AGE-REVERSING RULES FOR LIFE: SEVEN-STEP SUMMARY

By this point of the program, my patients tell me that they can't believe how much better they feel inside and out. Some of them even say they wouldn't have believed it in a million years until they tried it themselves. I giggle a bit when I hear my London patients tell me in their gorgeous British accents, "Annoyingly, I feel amazing: my mood is better, I've lost the 'food baby' [which is how they describe bloating], my skin has changed for the better; it's even toned, acne free, puffy free and my jowls even look lifted …" They can't believe their eyes. But before I go, I need to just add one final section—I don't want all these changes you've made to be fleeting, so let's wrap everything up with the seven steps I think help slow the rate of aging for life. Introduce these permanently into your life once you've finished all the plans, and you'll build on the anti-aging foundations now in place and reverse the signs of aging for good.

1) Live an 80:20 life

Unless you have a clear intolerance to one of the Ultimate Agers (see page 133), I suggest to my patients that once their gut is healed, 80 percent of their meals are free from gluten, sugar, dairy and alcohol, but if the other 20 percent of the time they want to consume them they should do so without guilt (guilt, like stress, is very aging). It might sound hard to reduce them like this for life now—temptation, after all, is everywhere—but the key is not to focus on what you need to avoid, but to look at all the foods you can have instead and choose your favorites. Then also think of these as choices that nourish your body and skin. If you think that way, why wouldn't you want to eat such foods? Nobody's perfect, and that 20 percent allows for this, but

I say to my patients that you won't know how good it feels to eat this way for life until you try it.

2) Listen to your body

Embrace Eastern, Western and naturopathic medicine. Each of us is unique and how much we need of anything in life depends on our own personal constitution. Your body is like a fine-tuned machine and it *will* tell you when something is wrong or if you're eating something that doesn't agree with you if you just listen. Its displeasure might manifest in clear symptoms in the gut, signs upon the skin or other health issues appearing elsewhere in the body. Using the face-mapping tips in Chapter 2 (see page 60) can also help you pinpoint any changes before they actually develop into symptoms. I recommend doing a regular face-mapping check once every few months just to see if there's anything you need to pay attention to.

3) Avoid eating processed foods

It's the easiest way to keep levels of inflammation down as you'll naturally lower your levels of omega-6, but it also limits chemical exposure. Every day we're learning more and more about what we're putting in our bodies and how it's impacting our health. As I was typing this chapter, a new study[10] came out that found two commonly used food additives (E466 and E433) directly damage the mucus that protects the gut. The closer to nature the food you eat, the better.

4) Variety is key

Don't stick to the same grains, fruits, vegetables or proteins all the time—the more varied your diet, the more nutrients you'll be taking in. On top of this, when someone is eating the same diet over and over again it can actually trigger a sensitivity to it. If, for example, you give up dairy but only ever drink almond milk, you could find you start to develop an intolerance to almonds. Rotating your diet is key to good health in many ways.

5) Eat seasonally

Our bodies are constantly on a cycle—we sleep and wake by one, our daily energy is controlled by one, our hormones have many cycles. The only constant is that things around us change! In terms of nutrition this means you should choose the food around that is freshest and therefore likely to be highest in nutrients, which means eating seasonally.

But there is also another element to eating seasonally that comes from Traditional Chinese Medicine (TCM), which is that we should eat foods that support the body's needs at any given time of year. Let me give you an example: in the winter it's generally cold and to warm us up we should reach for warming spices, hot meals and seasonal produce, such as root vegetables, that provide heat from within. This gives us an internal cozy blanket and fuels our "chi"—the internal energy that flows within us and that must remain balanced if we want to stay well. It also aids digestion as during winter we are in constriction mode where our blood vessels are closed, or blocked as we say in TCM, to keep in heat. Eat cold foods at that time and they stay closed, blood flow to the digestive system is reduced and you could find yourself getting bloated after meals. Eat warmer foods, however, and the vessels open. As digestion flows so does our chi. Conversely, during summer you should eat a cooler diet to counteract the heat that surrounds you. It's no coincidence that the foods in season around this time tend to be light and water filled—nature knows what our bodies need seasonally and attempts to provide it, if only we listen.

6) Eat mindfully

Chew your food well and slowly—doing so helps prevent digest-aging. Remember: chewing is the first step in digestion and doing it well will ensure you take in the maximum nutrients from the food you eat; nutrients that end up showing on your skin. Chewing well also has other benefits—it's been linked to more balanced levels of blood glucose and insulin, which helps reduce the aging impact of both of these on the system and makes you feel fuller faster. Those who eat slowly are less likely to develop gut-flammation than those who hurry their meals. As suggested on page 227, eat until you are 70–80 percent full. It takes about 20 minutes for your brain to realize that you are full, so if you stop at this point, you should be fully satisfied in a short while. Eat calmly and slowly while sitting at a table: the Italians do it right. They sit at the table for hours and enjoy the food they have in front of them. With eating should come pleasure. On which note, never eat when you are angry—it activates the sympathetic nervous system and causes the beginnings of digest-aging.

7) Live an anti-aging lifestyle

Remember the four rules: stress less, exercise moderately, sleep well and think youthful.

RECIPES

BREAKFASTS

CHIA PORRIDGE (serves 1)

> 2½ tbsp (25 g) chia seeds
> ¼ cup (60 ml) unsweetened nut milk (bought or homemade, see
>   page 260)
> 2 handfuls of berries of your choice
> 3 tbsp (25 g) crushed walnuts
> cinnamon to taste

1. Place the chia seeds in a bowl and add the nut milk. Stir and leave to stand for 5 minutes.
2. Stir again, being careful to smooth out any lumps. Leave for another 15 minutes until the seeds swell.
3. Add the berries and walnuts. Sprinkle with cinnamon and serve.

POWER PORRIDGES

All of these serve one and contain the same basic recipe—the preparation differs slightly by grain.

> ¼ cup (50 g) quinoa, amaranth or buckwheat flakes or groats
> ⅓–½ cup (75–125 ml) almond, coconut or hemp milk, depending
>   on taste
> 1–3 Superfood Power Ups of your choice (see page 235)

Superfood Power Ups

1 tsp maca powder

1 tsp acai puree

1 tsp cacao powder

1 tsp lucuma powder

1 tsp coconut oil or expeller-pressed coconut

1 tsp ground cinnamon

1 tsp chia seeds

1 tsp flaxseeds

1 tsp turmeric

1 tsp chlorella

1 tsp spirulina

1 tbsp nut butter

small handful of nuts

SWEET POTATO CAKES (makes 4)

14 oz/400 g (about 2 large) sweet potato, peeled
1 egg
1 tsp turmeric
1 tsp salt
freshly ground black pepper
2 tbsp olive oil

1. Grate the sweet potato using a cheese grater or a food processor with a grater attachment.
2. Whisk the egg in a large bowl, then add the sweet potato, turmeric and salt, and a grind of pepper.

3. Split the mixture into 4 and form patties using your hands.
4. Heat the oil in a frying pan over a medium heat and fry the patties for 2–3 minutes until they start to brown. Flip and fry for another 1–2 minutes.
5. You can freeze any unused patties. Defrost and fry on a low heat until they brown or grill them from frozen when you need to reuse.

BUCKWHEAT BIRCHER (serves 1)

¼ cup (50 g) buckwheat flakes or groats
½ tsp ground cinnamon
1 apple, chopped
½ cup plus 1 tbsp (150 ml) almond, coconut or hemp milk
1 handful of berries of your choice
1 oz (25 g) nuts of your choice

1. Add the buckwheat, cinnamon and apple to a bowl. Stir well, then add enough milk to just cover the mixture (you may not need all the milk), and leave in the fridge overnight to soak.
2. If you use groats and prefer a smoother texture, blend the soaked mixture.
3. Stir in the berries and nuts, then add a little more milk to thin if needed.

SMOOTH SKIN SMOOTHIE (serves 1)

7 fl oz (200 ml) nut milk
1–2 tbsp hemp, pea or rice protein powder
5 oz (150 g) frozen berries
½ banana
¼–½ avocado
small handful of baby spinach
3 mint leaves

1 tbsp chia seeds
1 tsp ground flaxseeds
pinch of ground cinnamon
Power Up: 1 tsp maca powder (optional)

Place everything into a blender or food processor and blend until smooth.

TURMERIC EGGS (serves 1)

3 eggs
1 tsp chia seeds
1 tsp turmeric
pinch of sea salt
2 tbsp coconut milk or coconut cream
2 tsp olive oil, divided
3½ oz (100 g) baby spinach
2 tbsp Super Skin Mix (see page 257)

1. Whisk the eggs, chia seeds, turmeric, sea salt and coconut milk in a bowl until combined, then set aside.
2. Pour 1 tsp of the olive oil into a frying pan over a low to medium heat.
3. Add the spinach and sauté gently for 30 seconds until wilted. Remove from the heat.
4. Add the remaining olive oil to a small saucepan and heat, then pour in the egg mixture and gently stir until the eggs are set but still creamy.
5. Add the spinach and Super Skin Mix and fold through.

LUNCHES

SPICY SOUP (serves 4)

> *2 pints (1.2 liters) Bone Broth (see page 239) or good-quality*
> *vegetable stock*
> *1 red chili, seeded and diced*
> *1 tbsp Thai fish sauce (optional)*
> *2 tbsp rice vinegar*
> *1 tbsp chili sauce*
> *3½ oz (100 g) baby chestnut mushrooms, finely sliced*
> *1 red bell pepper, finely sliced*
> *3½ oz (100 g) baby corn, finely sliced*
> *1 small carrot, finely sliced*
> *7 oz (200 g) soba or rice noodles*
> *7 oz (200 g) lean beef, cut into strips*
> *1 tsp chili oil*
> *2 tbsp chopped cilantro leaves*

1. Put the broth or stock into a large saucepan and add the chili, fish sauce, vinegar and chili sauce. Bring to a boil and simmer gently for 10 minutes.
2. Add the mushrooms, pepper, corn and carrot, and simmer for another 5 minutes, then add the noodles.
3. Stir in the beef strips and continue to simmer until cooked to your liking.
4. Ladle into 4 bowls and serve with a dash of chili oil and the cilantro. If taking this to work, place it in a thermos or Tupperware container and warm it at work.

Vegetarian version: Replace the beef with 8 oz (220 g) organic, non-GMO tofu, added in step 3 as above.

BONE BROTH (makes 5½–7 pints/3–4 liters)

*4½–6½ lb (2–3 kg) any bone (e.g., beef bones, chicken carcasses,
    fish bones, lamb bones or marrow bones)*
2 onions, chopped roughly
2 medium leeks
2 medium carrots
*small handful of bay leaves, parsley or mixed herbs (depending on
    preference)*
*Power Up: 1–2 tsp ground turmeric, for reducing gut-inflammation
    and a skin-friendly antioxidant boost (optional)*

1. Place all the ingredients in a large, heavy-bottomed saucepan.
2. Pour in enough water so the bones are covered, but leave some
   room at the top of the pan so the broth can bubble.
3. Bring to a boil and then turn down to a low heat. Simmer for 6–8
   hours for chicken carcasses or fish bones, and about 12 hours for
   other bones. Periodically check the water levels and scrape off any
   froth or foam that rises to the top.
4. Strain the liquid and either use immediately or store. Broth will
   store in a fridge for 3–4 days or you can freeze it in smaller portion
   sizes to make soups during the week.

MINTED QUINOA (serves 4)

5 oz (150 g) quinoa
4 ripe tomatoes, seeded and diced
1 small red onion, finely chopped
Himalayan salt and freshly ground black pepper

For the dressing:
juice of 2 lemons
½ oz (15 g) finely chopped mint leaves
2½ oz (75 g) cucumber, diced
2–3 tbsp olive or flaxseed oil
1 tsp Himalayan salt

1. Cook the quinoa as directed on the packet.
2. Meanwhile, prepare the dressing by simply mixing the lemon juice, mint, cucumber, oil, and Himalayan salt in a bowl.
3. Transfer the quinoa to a large bowl, add the dressing and stir with a fork until evenly mixed. Add the tomatoes and onion, then season to taste with the Himalayan salt and freshly ground black pepper.
4. If you're taking this to work you can keep the dressing separate and add it at the last minute if you prefer.

SEXY SKIN SALAD (serves 1)

3½–5 oz (100–150 g) boiled eggs or cooked chicken or beef or fish, or seafood or tofu or beans
1 handful of arugula
2 sticks of celery, chopped
1 tbsp pomegranate seeds
½ mango, diced
1 tbsp sunflower seeds
1 tbsp pumpkin seeds

1. Combine all the ingredients in a bowl and mix well.
2. Just before eating, add a serving of Skin-Boosting Salad Dressing (see page 257).

KALE AND APPLE SALAD (serves 1)

2 oz (50 g) new potatoes
½ tsp finely chopped mint leaves
4 oz (125 g) raw shelled prawns or shelled walnuts
coconut oil
3–4 handfuls of curly kale, finely chopped
2 oz (50 g) cashews
1 apple, unpeeled but cored and diced
1–2 tbsp pomegranate seeds

For the dressing:
2 tbsp fresh lemon juice
pinch of salt
1 very small garlic clove, puréed
1 tbsp extra-virgin olive oil
2 tbsp avocado

1. Cook the potatoes with the mint in a saucepan of boiling water for 10 minutes. Strain the potatoes and, when cool, halve them.
2. Stir-fry the prawns for 2–3 minutes in a little coconut oil until they turn pink.
3. Combine the potatoes and prawns (or walnuts) with the kale, cashews, apple and pomegranate seeds in a large bowl.
4. Combine all the dressing ingredients in a separate bowl using a hand blender.
5. Add the dressing to the salad and toss well. Leave to rest for 15 minutes—this softens the kale, which can be tough in salads if you leave it uncooked. If you're taking this to work, it will soften throughout the day.

CURRIED BRUSSELS SPROUTS SALAD (serves 4-6)

1 lb 2 oz (500 g) Brussels sprouts, sliced into halves or thirds
2 tsp olive oil
2 medium apples, cored and sliced
1 fennel bulb, finely sliced
4 spring onions, finely sliced
1 romaine lettuce, roughly chopped
2 oz (50 g) walnuts, chopped

For the dressing:
2 oz (50 g) raw cashews, soaked in cold water for 20 minutes
4 fl oz (120 ml) water
¾ oz (20 g) sultanas (golden raisins)

juice of ½ lemon
1 tsp curry powder
small handful of parsley leaves

1. Preheat the oven to 400°F/200°C/Gas Mark 6.
2. Tip the Brussels sprouts into a large oven tray in an even layer and stir through the oil. Roast for 15–20 minutes, until lightly browned. Set aside.
3. Meanwhile, combine the cashews, water, sultanas, lemon juice, curry powder and parsley for the dressing in a blender. Blend until completely smooth and creamy.
4. In a large bowl, combine the roasted Brussels sprouts, apple, fennel, spring onions, lettuce and walnuts. Drizzle over the salad dressing and serve.

DINNERS

VEGGIE BOWL (serves 1)

7 oz (200 g) mixed vegetables of your choice
1 tbsp olive oil
1 tsp mixed herbs
1½ oz (40 g) quinoa
1 serving of Lima Bean Hummus (see page 244)

1. Preheat the oven to 400°F/200°C/Gas Mark 6.
2. Chop the vegetables into large chunks and place in a roasting pan, drizzle with olive oil and add the herbs.
3. Roast in the oven for 45–60 minutes.
4. Cook the quinoa as directed on the packet then transfer it into the base of a bowl.
5. Add the hummus on top of the quinoa.
6. Serve with the vegetables on top.

STIR-FRY SKIN MAGIC

2 oz (50 g) brown rice
7 oz (200 g) mixed vegetables of your choice
dash of sesame or coconut oil
1 tbsp Harissa Mix (see page 258) (optional)
2 oz (50 g) cashews
1 tbsp kimchi or Chili Power (see page 256) (optional)

1. Cook the rice as directed on the packet.
2. Stir-fry all the vegetables in a little sesame or coconut oil (with the Harissa Mix, if using).
3. Add the cashews and toss briefly to warm.
4. Serve on top of the rice with kimchi or Chili Power, if using.

PREBIOTIC POWER BOWL

2 oz (50 g) brown or green lentils
2–3 tbsp Bone Broth (see page 239) or good-quality stock
3–4 spears of asparagus, chopped
1 leek, chopped
½ red bell pepper, chopped
3½ oz (100 g) broccoli
1 oz (25 g) pine nuts
1–2 tsp coconut oil
1 serving of Skin-Boosting Salad Dressing (see page 257)

1. Boil the lentils in the bone broth as directed on the packet.
2. In the meantime, stir-fry the asparagus, leek, pepper, broccoli and pine nuts in coconut oil.
3. Transfer the lentils to a plate, and drizzle with the dressing.
4. Place all the vegetables on top and serve.

LIMA BEAN HUMMUS (makes 2–3 servings)

14 oz (400 g) can of lima beans
juice of 1 lemon
1 tbsp tahini
2 tbsp olive oil
1 tsp ground cumin
1 tsp coriander seeds
salt and freshly ground black pepper

1. Drain the beans in a sieve and rinse with water.
2. Add to a food processor with the S-blade attachment.
3. Add the lemon juice, tahini, olive oil, cumin and coriander seeds.
4. Blend. Taste and add more lemon and/or cumin if needed. If it's too thick, add 1 tbsp of water and continue to blend. Season to taste with salt and pepper.
5. Transfer to a lidded glass jar and put in the fridge. It will keep for 3–4 days.

Variation: Replace the lima beans with chickpeas. For a creamier hummus, add more olive oil—up to 3 more tablespoons.

SPICED LENTILS (serves 4)

8 oz (225 g) Puy or brown lentils
2 bay leaves
2 tsp cumin seeds
1 tbsp olive oil
1 small onion, chopped
2 celery sticks, chopped
2 carrots, chopped
juice of ½ lemon
salt and pepper
4–5 celery leaves, shredded

1. Rinse the lentils well, then transfer to a saucepan of cold water and bring to a boil. Skim the surface, then add the bay leaves and simmer for 20–25 minutes, until just soft.
2. Meanwhile, place the cumin seeds in a frying pan over a medium heat, shaking the pan until they release their fragrance. Immediately add the olive oil, along with the onion, celery and carrots. Cook, stirring frequently, for 6–7 minutes.
3. Drain the lentils and toss into the fried vegetables. Add the lemon juice, season generously with salt and pepper and stir in the celery leaves.

HEALTHY CURRY (serves 4)

½ tsp coconut oil
2 tsp turmeric
2 tsp ground cumin
1–2 green chilies, finely chopped
2 tbsp tomato paste
2 tbsp crushed fresh ginger
1 lb 2 oz (500 g) sweet potatoes, peeled and cut into small chunks
2 large carrots, peeled and cut into small chunks
14 fl oz (400 ml) coconut milk
14 oz (400 g) chopped tomatoes
½ cauliflower, chopped
14 oz (400 g) ready-to-eat beans of your choice, e.g., chickpeas
7 oz (20 g) brown or wild rice or quinoa
3 cardamom pods
2 cinnamon sticks
2 pinches of saffron
14 oz (400 g) raw prawns
7 oz (200 g) baby spinach, washed and drained
juice of 1 lime
handful of cilantro leaves, roughly chopped

1. Heat the oil in a large heavy-bottomed saucepan and, when hot, add the turmeric, cumin, chilies, tomato paste and ginger. Fry gently for 2 minutes until fragrant.
2. Stir in the sweet potatoes, carrots, coconut milk and chopped tomatoes, and simmer for 15 minutes before adding the cauliflower and your choice of beans. Simmer for another 5 minutes, until all of the vegetables are tender.
3. Meanwhile, cook the brown or wild rice or quinoa in a separate saucepan, along with the cardamom, cinnamon sticks and saffron, according to the packet.
4. Stir the prawns and spinach through the curry, and simmer for 2–3 more minutes until the prawns turn opaque and are cooked through.
5. Remove the cinnamon sticks from the rice or quinoa and divide it between 4 plates. Spoon the curry over the rice, then sprinkle the lime juice and cilantro on top.

BUTTERNUT SQUASH SOUP (serves 4)

2 tbsp olive oil
1 large leek, thickly sliced
1 celery stick, chopped
1 garlic clove, chopped
1 tbsp chopped sage leaves
1 small red chili, halved and seeded
1 lb (450 g) butternut squash, peeled, seeded and diced (you need about 12 oz/350 g of flesh)
1¾ pint (1 liter) Bone Broth (see page 239) or good-quality vegetable stock
pinch of cayenne pepper
8 oz (200 g) cooked lima beans
salt and pepper

1. Heat the oil in a large saucepan, then add the leek, celery and garlic, and fry over a low heat for 10 minutes. Add the sage, chili and squash, and stir-fry for 5 minutes until the squash begins to color.
2. Pour in the broth or stock, add the cayenne, increase the heat and bring to a boil. Cover and simmer for 35 minutes.
3. Transfer to a food processor and blend until smooth. Return to the pan, add the beans and heat through. Season with salt and pepper to taste.

MEXICAN PEPPERS (serves 4)

3 onions, peeled and halved vertically with the root end still attached
2–3 hot chilies, seeded and sliced
2 garlic cloves, crushed
2 tbsp chopped cilantro leaves
zest and juice of 2 limes
1 lb 5 oz (600 g) skinless chicken breasts
1–2 tbsp olive oil
6 mixed red, yellow or orange bell peppers, cored and cut into wedges
salt and pepper

1. Cut each half of the onions into wedges, working from the root end to the top but making sure each wedge is still held together at the root end.
2. Put the onions, chilies, garlic, cilantro and lime zest and juice into a large shallow dish and mix thoroughly. Cut the chicken into large pieces and add to the dish. Stir well, cover and leave to marinate in the fridge for at least 1 hour or overnight, if possible.
3. Heat the oil in a heavy-bottomed frying pan. Remove the chicken and onions from the marinade with a slotted spoon and add them to the pan, reserving the marinade. Fry over a high heat for around 5 minutes, turning occasionally, until the chicken is thoroughly browned on the outside. Remove the chicken from the pan and set aside.

4. Add the peppers to the pan and cook for about 5 minutes, stirring occasionally, until the onions and peppers have softened.
5. Return the chicken to the pan, add the marinade, lower the heat and cook for about 5 more minutes, stirring occasionally, until the chicken is cooked through. Serve with cooked brown or wild rice.

Vegetarian version: Omit the chicken from the recipe and instead of returning the chicken to the pan in step 5, add 1 lb 2 oz (500 g) cooked, rinsed black beans along with the marinade and heat through for 5 minutes.

CHICKPEAS WITH SPINACH (serves 4)

15 oz (425 g) can of chickpeas
1–2 tbsp ghee
½ in (1 cm) piece fresh ginger, chopped
1–2 garlic cloves, crushed
1 tsp ground coriander
½ tsp ground cumin
1 tsp paprika
2 tomatoes, finely chopped
8 oz (225 g) spinach, chopped
small handful of cilantro leaves, roughly torn
salt and freshly ground black pepper

1. Drain the chickpeas and rinse them under cold water.
2. Heat the ghee in a large heavy-bottomed saucepan. Add the ginger, garlic, ground coriander, cumin and paprika, and cook for 2 minutes, stirring all the time. Pour in the chickpeas and stir to coat in the spice mixture.

3. Add the tomatoes, spinach and cilantro leaves, then cook for 2 minutes. Cover with a lid and simmer gently for 10 minutes. Season with salt and pepper before serving.

STUFFED PEPPERS (serves 4)

5 oz (150 g) quinoa or buckwheat
1–2 tbsp coconut oil
1 tsp sea salt
¾ tsp freshly ground black pepper
2 tbsp paprika
4 garlic cloves, chopped
1 medium onion, chopped
2 celery stalks, chopped
1 lb 2 oz (500 g) broccoli, chopped
4 red bell peppers
juice of ½ lemon
handful of flat leaf parsley, roughly chopped

1. Preheat the oven to 350°F/180°C/Gas Mark 4.
2. Cook the quinoa or buckwheat according to the packet, then set aside.
3. Heat the coconut oil in a large frying pan and, when hot, add the salt, pepper, paprika, garlic, onion, celery and broccoli. Cook gently for 8–10 minutes, until the onion is soft and translucent and the vegetables are tender.
4. Add the quinoa or buckwheat to the pan and mix well.
5. Halve the peppers, remove the core and seeds, then fill each half with an eighth of the cooked mixture.
6. Put the stuffed peppers into a large oiled baking dish and bake for 45 minutes. Sprinkle the lemon juice and parsley over them to serve.

SPICED NOODLE SOUP (serves 4)

2 skinless chicken thighs, on the bone
2 lemongrass stalks, finely sliced
2-in (5-cm) piece fresh ginger, sliced
2 red chilies, sliced
2 garlic cloves, sliced
3½ oz (100 g) soba or rice noodles
2 carrots, cut into matchsticks
6 stems broccolini or Chinese broccoli, roughly chopped
½ red bell pepper, cut into strips
3½ oz (100 g) bean sprouts
2 tbsp gluten-free miso paste
2 tsp sesame oil
2 spring onions, finely sliced, to garnish

1. Put the chicken, lemongrass, ginger, chili and garlic into a large, lidded saucepan with 1 pint (600 ml) of water. Cover and bring to a boil. Reduce the heat and simmer for 20 minutes.
2. Lift the chicken out of the pan using a slotted spoon and put it on a cutting board. Strain the stock into another large saucepan, discard the leftover spices and add ½ pint (300 ml) of water. Shred the chicken and set to one side.
3. Bring the strained stock up to a boil and add the noodles, carrots and broccoli. Simmer for 3 minutes.
4. Return the chicken to the stock, add the pepper and bean sprouts and stir in the miso paste. Simmer for another minute until the chicken is heated through and the vegetables are tender.
5. Ladle between 4 bowls, stir in the sesame oil and sprinkle with the spring onion.

Vegetarian version: Omit the chicken. At step 4, add 200 g firm tofu and simmer for 3–5 minutes to heat through.

COD PROVENÇALE (serves 4)

4 x 5 oz (150 g) cod fillets
2½ fl oz (75 ml) olive oil
1 onion, finely chopped
1 tsp dried oregano
3 garlic cloves, chopped
14 oz (400 g) can of peeled plum tomatoes
1 tbsp tomato paste
salt and pepper
12 small black olives

1. Rinse the fish and pat dry with paper towels; set aside.
2. Heat the olive oil in a large shallow frying pan with a lid, which will be needed later. Add the onion and oregano, and cook over a very low heat for 10 minutes, stirring frequently.
3. Add the garlic and fry for another 2–3 minutes until the onion is translucent and beginning to turn pale golden.
4. Stir in the tomatoes, mashing them with a fork to break them down. Mix in the tomato paste. Bring the sauce to a boil. Season with salt and pepper to taste.
5. Bury the fish fillets in the tomato sauce and scatter the olives between them. Cover the pan and simmer gently for 6 minutes, then turn the fish over and continue cooking for another 4–5 minutes, until you can just pull the flesh from the bone with the tip of a knife.

CAULIFLOWER PIZZA (makes one 12 in/30 cm pizza)

For the base:
1 large cauliflower, about 1½ lb (700 g), trimmed and cut into chunks
3½ oz (100 g) ground almonds
2 tbsp nutritional yeast
2 medium eggs, beaten
salt and freshly ground black pepper

For the topping:
1 tsp olive oil
1 small onion, finely chopped
1 garlic clove, crushed
9 oz (250 g) tomato purée
1 tbsp tomato paste
1 large zucchini, roughly sliced
1 red bell pepper, finely sliced
5 oz (150 g) asparagus, roughly chopped, woody ends discarded
3 sun-dried tomatoes, roughly chopped
1 chicken breast, cooked and shredded
handful of basil leaves

1. Preheat the oven to 400°F/200°C/Gas Mark 6.
2. Steam the cauliflower for 3–4 minutes, until just tender. Leave to steam dry for a few minutes before blitzing in a food processor until it reaches a rice-like consistency.
3. Tip the cauliflower into a sieve and place over a bowl. Press down on the cauliflower with the back of a spoon repeatedly until you have pushed as much liquid out of the cauliflower as possible. Transfer to a large clean bowl.

4. Stir in the ground almonds, nutritional yeast and eggs, and season with a little salt and pepper.

5. Line a large baking sheet with parchment and spoon the cauliflower mixture into the middle. Use the back of a spoon and your fingertips to flatten out the "dough" into a 12 in (30 cm) round pizza base.

6. Bake in the oven for 12–15 minutes, until golden brown. Set aside.

7. Meanwhile, heat the oil in a large frying pan and add the onion. Fry gently for 4–5 minutes, until softened, before adding the garlic. Cook, stirring, for another minute, until fragrant.

8. Pour the tomato purée and paste into the pan and simmer for 6–8 minutes, until the sauce has thickened. Season with a little salt and pepper.

9. While the sauce is cooking place the zucchini, pepper and asparagus on to a lightly oiled baking tray and roast for 6–8 minutes, until lightly golden.

10. Spread the sauce on to the pizza base until it almost reaches the edges, and sprinkle the roasted vegetables, sun-dried tomatoes and chicken breast on top.

11. Return the pizza to the oven for 8–10 minutes, until the pizza is golden and crisp at the edges. Scatter with the basil leaves and serve in slices.

CHILI AND CAULIFLOWER RICE (serves 4–6)

4 tbsp olive oil, divided
1 red onion, finely chopped
3 garlic cloves, crushed
2–3 dried hot red chilies, crumbled
1 tbsp mild paprika
1 tbsp tomato paste
2 tsp cumin seeds
2 bay leaves
1 cinnamon stick
8 oz (230 g) ready-to-eat red kidney beans
8 oz (230 g) ready-to-eat black-eyed peas
about 1½ lb (700 g) of mixed vegetables (carrots, peppers, eggplant),
   cut into chunks
14 oz (400 g) chopped tomatoes
1 large handful of cilantro
salt and pepper

For the Cauliflower Rice:
1 medium cauliflower
olive oil or coconut oil

1. Heat half the oil in a large saucepan. Add the onion, half the garlic and half the chili. Cook, stirring regularly, for 5 minutes until the onion softens.
2. Add the paprika, tomato paste, cumin seeds and cook, stirring, for 2 minutes.
3. Add the bay leaves, cinnamon stick, beans and prepared vegetables and stir for 2 minutes.
4. Add the tomatoes and about 5 fl oz (150 ml) of water and bring to a boil.
5. Simmer for 45 minutes to 1 hour until the vegetables are tender.
6. If the mixture begins to stick, add more water.

7. While the chili cooks, remove the outer leaves from the cauliflower, cut into chunks and run through a food processor with a grater blade.

8. Ten minutes before the chili is ready, add a little olive oil or coconut oil to a large pan with a lid. Throw in the cauliflower rice and stir well. Place the lid and cook on a low heat for 5–8 minutes. It should be al dente for best results.

9. Serve the chili on the cauliflower rice and top with cilantro.

DIPS AND MIXES

BASIC NUT BUTTER (makes 10 servings)

10½ oz (300 g) any unsalted, unroasted nut (e.g., cashews, peanuts, almonds or walnuts)

1. Put all the nuts in a food processor with the S-blade attachment.

2. Blend until you have a creamy butter. Exactly how long you will need to blend for will depend on the nuts. The oilier they are, the faster you'll create the butter—peanuts take a relatively quick 4–5 minutes, cashews and almonds may take 20–30 minutes depending on how powerful your food processor is. You'll start with chopped nuts, progress to a mix that looks like flour, then on to what looks like dough—and eventually a creamy butter.

3. Turn the food processor off periodically and scrape down the sides to ensure all the chopped nuts are mixed in. As you do this, you can also add chili, cinnamon or turmeric to give an extra beauty boost. For a nut that takes more than 5 minutes you might also want to give your food processor a few minutes break in between sessions to let it cool.

4. The longer a nut takes to process the drier the butter will be. If you want a smoother butter, try soaking the nuts for 20–30 minutes before blending, or add 1–2 tbsp of coconut oil at the end of the process.

5. The butter will be warm when you finish, so spoon it into an airtight jar and allow to cool in the fridge before eating. It will keep for up to 2 weeks in the fridge.

PERFECT SKIN DIP (makes 2–3 servings)

1 avocado, peeled and pitted
1 oz (20 g) finely diced onion or shallot
juice of 1 lime
½ tbsp cold pressed olive or avocado oil
pinch of sea salt
pinch of ground black or white pepper
small handful of cilantro leaves

1. Chop the avocado into rough chunks.
2. Transfer into a food processor along with the onion, lime juice, oil, sea salt and pepper.
3. Blend to your preferred consistency. Add the cilantro, pulse briefly to combine, and serve.
4. Store any left over in an airtight container in the fridge. It will last 3–4 days.

CHILI POWER SPICY SAUCE (add to salads, chicken or fish dishes for an extra kick)

3–4 large green chilies (roughly chopped and seeded for a less spicy sauce)
juice of 2 large lemons
½ tsp Himalayan salt
1 garlic clove
1 tbsp extra virgin olive oil
3 oz (80 g) fresh cilantro

Put all the ingredients into a small bowl and blend with a hand blender until smooth. It will last 3–4 days in the fridge or you can freeze it in ice cube trays and defrost when needed.

SUPER SKIN MIX (makes 3–4 servings)

large bunch of parsley
large bunch of basil
1 clove garlic, crushed
1–2 tbsp lemon juice
½ tsp freshly ground black pepper
¼ tsp sea salt
2–3 tbsp olive oil

1. Put the parsley, basil and garlic into a food processor and blend until the herbs are finely chopped.
2. Add lemon juice, pepper, salt and olive oil.
3. Blend again until you have a lovely green fragrant paste.

SKIN-BOOSTING SALAD DRESSING (makes 5 servings)

3 tbsp olive or flaxseed oil
2 tbsp apple cider vinegar
juice of ½ lemon
1–2 pinches of turmeric
pinch of sea salt
freshly ground black pepper

Place all the ingredients in a jar, put on the lid and shake well.

MUSTARD DRESSING (makes 4 servings)

6 tsp olive oil
4 tsp apple cider vinegar
1 tsp gluten-free mustard
1 tsp chili powder
15 mint leaves, finely chopped
2 sprigs of dill, finely chopped

Place all the ingredients in a jar, put on the lid and shake well. Store in the fridge for up to 1 week.

HARISSA MIX (makes 8–10 servings)

10–12 dried red chili peppers
3 cloves garlic, minced
½ tsp salt
2 tbsp olive oil, plus extra to preserve
1 tsp ground coriander
1 tsp ground caraway seeds
½ tsp ground cumin

1. Soak the dried chilies in a bowl of hot water for 30 minutes. Drain. Remove and discard the stems and seeds.
2. Put the rehydrated chilies, along with the garlic, salt and oil into a food processor. Blend into a smooth paste.
3. Add remaining spices and process until combined.
4. Transfer to an airtight container. Drizzle a small amount of olive oil on top of the paste to keep it fresh. This will keep for up to 1 month in the refrigerator.

JUICES AND MILKS

GREEN JUICES (serves 1)

Juices based around vegetables can be an acquired taste, so if you aren't used to drinking them gradually work up to stronger versions. To make these juices you will need a real juicer rather than a blender.

For Beginners: Skin Softener Greens

2 apples, halved
1 cucumber
3 large handfuls of spinach
2 lemons, peeled
small handful of mint leaves

Wash everything well. Place all the ingredients into a juicer and juice. Serve immediately.

Moving On Up: Green Age Reversal

1 peach, pitted
½ cucumber
2 handfuls of kale
handful of spinach
1 lemon, peeled

Wash everything well. Juice all the ingredients in a juicer, and serve immediately.

For Absolute Devotees: Flawless

5 kale leaves
small handful of parsley
1 apple
1 pear
1 lime
1 cucumber
2 celery sticks
½–¾ in (1–2 cm) piece fresh ginger, peeled
1 tsp spirulina or chlorella

Wash all of the ingredients well, then juice everything in a juicer. Serve immediately.

NUT MILKS (makes 1 liter/2 pints)

3½ oz (100 g) raw, blanched almonds or raw cashews
pinch of stevia
1 liter (2 pints) of water

1. Place all the ingredients into a blender and blend on a high speed until smooth.
2. Use the milk as it is if using in desserts or with cereal, or strain through a sieve if you want a true "milk" texture. Store in an airtight container in the fridge for up to 4 days.

COCONUT MILK (makes 150 ml)

2 oz (50 g) fresh coconut flesh, grated

1. Put the fresh coconut into a small glass jar and place this in hot water for 10 minutes. It will become semi-liquid, which makes it easier to mix without lumps forming in the milk. If you have a hand blender you can skip this stage and simply use the blender to smooth out any lumps.

2. Now add 5 fl oz (150 ml) of water. Mix well.

If you want to make a larger quantity, follow the same method and use three parts water to every one part coconut. To make a thicker, creamier consistency milk, use two parts coconut to every three parts water. The milk will keep in the fridge for up to 3 days.

AFTERWORD

It takes a short while from when you type the last few lines of a book to the day and the moment we're at now, where you're holding the finished copy in your hand. I'm writing this somewhere in between all those points and it seems that almost daily a new study or one of my peers is discussing a new finding regarding the importance of one of the subjects in this book. They're linking inflammation to depression, and research in gut health has shown even more links between the importance of the microbiome in weight control and how much we worry. Things are moving so fast it's hard to keep up—and yet I think we're still only at the start of learning about this incredible field.

I'm certain that the idea that "everything starts in the gut" is simply going to develop and grow as our understanding of the impact and interrelation of the microbiome, the digestive system, inflammation and hormones on how fast, and how healthily, we age both inside and out also develops and grows. Scientists are already talking about how diets in the future will be specifically tailored to ensure they help us create the perfect mix of bacteria for our bodies—and I'm proud that, in a way, I'm helping you get in on the ground level of embracing what could quite literally become the future of modern medicine.

You might have bought this book as a way simply to reverse the physical signs of aging, but I'm hoping that the more you have read, the more you realize it's so much more than that. That, in fact, it's as likely to make you feel amazing as look incredible, and that you now have at your disposal an entire toolbox that helps you fight aging and stay healthy for as long as you possibly can. I really do hope you're as excited as I am by what this might do for you now and in the future, and I'd love to hear how you get on. You'll find me on Twitter at @drnigma and on Instagram @drnigmatalib.

APPENDIX
PUTTING IT ALL INTO PRACTICE— YOUR 12-WEEK PLAN

One thing you might be wondering as you read through the plans is how you put everything together; it's actually pretty simple if you think of it as a stage-by-stage, step-by-step process.

STAGE 1: HEALTHY GUT

Weeks 1 and 2: Clear

- Follow the Age-Reversing Eating Plan to remove gluten, dairy, sugar and alcohol—this also implements all the dietary suggestions for all the plans unless specifically mentioned.
- Take the steps in the Clear plan.
- Reduce pesticide exposure with the organic eating rules.
- Start to work on managing stress.
- Identify any intolerances or sensitivities using the advice in Chapter 2.
- If you are in pain, try natural alternatives to painkillers.
- Consider having a stool test.

Week 3: Correct

- Introduce a quality probiotic to your diet.
- Chew better, try digestive bitters or supplement with Betaine HCl and pepsin.
- Take a digestive enzyme supplement.

Week 4: Protect
Add any gut-supporting supplements from the below:

- DGL: 1–3 tablets of 380–400 mg daily.
- Mastic gum: 1,000 mg, 1–2 times daily.
- Aloe vera: 1 glass of juice daily.
- Glutamine: 1,000–1,500 mg daily.
- Slippery elm: 400–500 mg, 3–4 times daily.

Time to assess
One you've reached this point, you are well on the path to healing your gut (and fighting aging from within). You can keep going for a few weeks longer following the plan as it stands now or, if you think you're making good progress (retake the digest-aging questionnaire on page 9 to help measure this), then it's time to start the Inflammation-Fighting CCP Plan.

STAGE 2: PUTTING OUT THE FIRE WITHIN
Weeks 5 and 6: Clear
- Keep following the Age-Reversing Eating Plan as it integrates all the diet advice recommended in this plan, but start to make your own meals if you haven't already.
- Reduce inflammatory triggers.
- Start addressing any inflammatory health concerns.
- Check your weight.
- Start doing some moderate exercise if you don't already.
- Work on improving sleep.
- Keep working on managing stress.

Week 7: Correct
- Introduce a fish oil—1,000 mg daily—or echium oil (as directed).

Week 8: Protect

Add one of the bad enzyme blockers if you're using them:

- GLA: 500 mg, 2 times daily.
- Boswellia: 300 mg, 3 times daily.
- Pycnogenol: 1 mg per kilogram (2.2 pounds) you weigh.

Time to assess

You can repeat the digest-aging questionnaire again, but this is also a good time to check that photograph I suggested you took. You should now see a clear difference—blemishes should be reduced or eliminated, skin texture smoother, tone more even and your fine lines and wrinkles softer. You will see a glow to the skin that sparkles from within.

STAGE 3: BALANCING YOUR HORMONES

Weeks 9 and 10: Clear

- Again, follow the Age-Reversing Eating Plan as it integrates the main dietary rules of this part of the plan.
- Reduce chemical exposure by:
  » Using a water filter.
  » Swapping to chemical-free cleaning products.
  » Choosing more natural beauty products.
  » Taking 500–1,000 mg of calcium d-glucarate, if using. (See contradictions on page 135.)
  » This is also an excellent time to start integrating all the beauty tips from Chapter 5 if you haven't done so already— by now, your skin will be reaping all the benefits of your internal makeover and be extremely responsive to a good skincare regime.

Week 11: Correct

- Keep working on improving sleep, managing stress and exercising appropriately.
- Consider having a hormone profile test.
- Start taking a hormone-balancing supplement, if using:
  - » Maca: 3–9 g daily.
  - » Chasteberry extract: 200 mg daily.
  - » Black cohosh: 6.5 mg of extract daily.
  - » Relora: as directed.
  - » DIM: 100–300 mg daily.
  - » L'Arginine: 5–9 g daily.
  - » Fenugreek: 2.5 g, 2 times daily.
  - » Bittermelon: 100–200 mg daily.

Week 12: Protect

- Add milk thistle, if using, 200–250 mg of standardized extract, three times a day.
- Book a sauna or steam three times a week (or exercise hard enough to sweat).
- Add one or two portions of isoflavone-heavy foods such as fermented soy, tofu, peanuts and alfalfa to the menu daily. This isn't in the plan as it stands as not everyone will need to eat them.

STAGE 4

Follow the tips to reverse aging for life from now on to consolidate all the amazing changes you've made. I hope you're now inspired to take control over your own destiny to improve the health of your skin and your body as a whole.

Note: if you are extending the Clear part of any plan for longer than a week then this whole plan will take a little longer than 12 weeks. That's no problem; keep doing things in turn, just accounting for the extra days you spent in those first vital stages.

SOURCES AND REFERENCES

Introduction
Association of Accredited Naturopathic Medical Colleges

Chapter 1
1   Helander H. F. and Fändriks L. "Surface area of the digestive tract—revisited." *Scandinavian Journal of Gastroenterology* June 2014; 49(6): 681–9
2   Volkova L. A., Khalif I. L. and Kabanova I. N. "Impact of the impaired intestinal microflora on the course of acne vulgaris." *Klinicheskaia Meditsina* 2001; 79(6): 39–41
3   Messaoudi M., et al. "Assessment of psychotropic-like properties of a probiotic formulation (Lactobacillus helveticus R0052 and Bifidobacterium longum R0175) in rats and human subjects." *British Journal of Nutrition* March 2011; 105(5): 755–64
4   Guyuron B., et al. "Factors contributing to the facial aging of identical twins." *Plastic and Reconstructive Surgery* April 2009; 123(4): 1321–31
5   Laugier R., Bernard J. P., Berthezene P. and Dupuy P. "Changes in pancreatic exocrine secretion with age: pancreatic exocrine secretion does decrease in the elderly." *Digestion* 1991; 50(3–4): 202–11
6   Le Chatelier E., et al. "Richness of human gut microbiome correlates with metabolic markers." *Nature* August 29, 2013; 500(7464): 541–6
7   David L. A., et al. "Diet rapidly and reproducibly alters the human gut microbiome." *Nature* January 23, 2014; 505(7484): 559–63
8   Bailey M. T., et al. "Exposure to a social stressor alters the structure of the intestinal microbiota: implications for stressor-induced

immunomodulation." *Brain, Behavior Immunity* March 2011; 25(3): 397–407

9   Dethlefsen L. and Relman D. A. "Incomplete recovery and individualized responses of the human distal gut microbiota to repeated antibiotic perturbation." *Proceedings of the National Academy of Sciences of the United States of America* Mar 15, 2011; 108, suppl 1: 4554–61

10 Peguet-Navarro J., et al. "Supplementation with oral probiotic bacteria protects human cutaneous immune homeostatis after UV exposure: double blind, randomized, placebo controlled clinical trial." *European Journal of Dermatology* September–October 2008; 18(5): 504–11

11 Benyacoub J., et al. "Immune modulation property of Lactobacillus paracasei NCC2461 (ST11) strain and impact on skin defenses." *Beneficial Microbes* June 1, 2014; 5(2): 129–36

12 Puch F., et al. "Consumption of functional fermented milk containing borage oil, green tea and vitamin E enhances skin barrier function." *Experimental Dermatology* August 2008; 17(8): 668–74

13 Kappus K. K., Juranek D. D. and Roberts J. M. "Results of testing for intestinal parasites by state diagnostic laboratories, United States, 1987." *CDC Surveillance Summaries: Morbidity and Mortality Weekly Report* December 1991; 40(4): 25–45

14 Franklin M. "The real causes of IBS: how they can be revealed by comprehensive digestive stool analysis." *Positive Health* March 2006; 121

15 Celiac UK. "About celiac disease and dermatitis herpetiformis" [online] www.celiac.org.uk

16 Rubio-Tapia A., et al. "The prevalence of celiac disease in the United States." *American Journal of Gastroenterology* October 2012; 107(10): 1538–44

Chapter 2

1   Fink B., Grammer K. and Matts P. J. "Visible skin color distribution plays a role in the perception of age, attractiveness and health in female faces." *Evolution and Human Behavior* November 2006; 27(6): 433–442

2   Dyer D. G., et al. "Accumulation of Maillard reaction products in skin collagen in diabetes and aging." *Journal of Clinical Investigation* June 1993; 91(6): 2463–9

3   Mayo Clinic. "Celiac Disease: On the Rise." *Discovery's Edge* July 2010; [online] www.mayo.edu

4   Zanini B., et al. "Search for atoxic cereals: a single blind, cross-over study on the safety of a single dose of Triticum monococcum, in patients with celiac disease." *BMC Gastroenterology* 2013; 13: 92

5   Ho S., Woodford K., Kukuljan S. and Pal S. "Comparative effects of A1 versus A2 beta-casein on gastrointestinal measures: a blinded randomised cross-over pilot study." *European Journal of Clinical Nutrition* September 2014; 68(9): 994–1000

6   Sapone A., et al. "Divergence of gut permeability and mucosal immune gene expression in two gluten-associated conditions: celiac disease and gluten sensitivity." *BMC Medicine* March 2011: 23

7   Adebamowo C. A., et al. "High school dietary dairy intake and teenage acne." *Journal of the American Academy of Dermatology* February 2005; 52(2): 207–14

8   Corder, R. et al. "Oenology: red wine procyanidins and vascular health." *Nature* November 30, 2006; 444 (7119): 566

9   Choi Y. K., et al. "Fructose intolerance: an under-recognized problem." *American Journal of Gastroenterology* June 2003; 98(6): 1348–53

Chapter 3

1   Thornfeldt C. R. "Chronic inflammation is etiology of extrinsic aging." *Journal of Cosmetic Dermatology* March 2008; 7(1): 78–82

2   Antvorskov J. C., Fundova P., Buschard K. and Funda D. P. "Dietary gluten alters the balance of pro-inflammatory and anti-inflammatory cytokines in T cells of BALB/c mice." *Immunology* January 2013; 138(1): 23–33

3   Labonté M. È., et al. "Impact of dairy products on biomarkers of inflammation: a systematic review of randomized controlled nutritional intervention studies in overweight and obese adults." *American Journal of Clinical Nutrition* April 2013; 97(4): 706–17

4   Dickinson S., et al. "High-glycemic index carbohydrate increases nuclear factor-kappaB activation in mononuclear cells of young, lean healthy subjects." *American Journal of Clinical Nutrition* May 2008; 87(5): 1188–93

5   Leung C. W., et al. "Soda and cell aging: associations between sugar-sweetened beverage consumption and leukocyte telomere length in healthy adults from the National Health and Nutrition Examination Surveys." *American Journal of Public Health* December 2014; 104(12): 2425–31

6   Clapp J., Curtis C. J., Middleton A. E. and Goldstein G. P. "Prevalence of partially hydrogenated oils in US packaged foods, 2012." *Preventing Chronic Disease* 2014; 11: 140–161

7   Visser M., et al. "Elevated C-reactive protein levels in overweight and obese adults." *Journal of the American Medical Association* December 8, 1999; 282(22): 2131–5

8   Deng T., et al. "Class II major histocompatibility complex plays an essential role in obesity-induced adipose inflammation." *Cell Metabolism* March 5, 2013; 17(3): 411–22

9   Zoccola P. M., et al. "Differential effects of post stressor rumination and distraction on cortisol and C-reactive protein." *Health Psychology* December 2014; 33(12): 1606–9

10   Cohen S., et al. "Chronic stress, glucocorticoid receptor resistance, inflammation and disease risk." *Proceedings of the National Academy of Sciences of the USA* April 17, 2012; 109(16): 5995–9

11   Morris A., et al. "Sleep quality and duration are associated with higher levels of inflammatory biomarkers: the META-Health Study." Presented at the American Heart Association 2010 Scientific Sessions, Chicago

12   Okada H. C. "Facial changes caused by smoking: a comparison between smoking and non-smoking identical twins." *Plastic and Reconstructive Surgery* November 2013; 132(5): 1085–92

13   Yates T., et al. "Self-reported sitting time and markers of inflammation, insulin resistance and adiposity." *American Journal of Preventive Medicine* January 2012; 42(1): 1–7

14   León-Latre M., et al. "Sedentary lifestyle and its relation to cardiovascular risk factors, insulin resistance and inflammatory

profile." *Revista Española Cardiología* (English Edition) June 2014; 67(6): 449–55

15 Adler A. S., et al. "Motif module map reveals enforcement of aging by continual NF-kappaB activity." *Genes and Development* December 15, 2007; 21(24): 3244–57

16 Imayama I., et al. "Effects of a caloric restriction weight loss diet and exercise on inflammatory biomarkers in overweight/obese postmenopausal women: a randomized controlled trial." *Cancer Research* May 1, 2012; 72(9): 2314–26

17 Health & Social Care Information Centre. "Statistics on obesity, physical activity and diet (England) 2014" [online] www.hscis.gov.uk

18 National Obesity Forum. "State of the Nation's Waistline 2015." December 2014; [online] www.nationalobesityforum.org.uk

19 Kiecolt-Glaser J. K., et al. "Omega-3 supplementation lowers inflammation and anxiety in medical students: a randomized controlled trial." *Brain, Behaviour and Immunity* November 2011; 25(8): 1725–34

20 Bradbury J., Myers S. P., and Oliver C. "An adaptogenic role for omega-3 fatty acids in stress: a randomised placebo controlled double blind intervention study (pilot)." *Nutrition Journal* November 28, 2004; 3: 20

21 Aggarwal B. B. and Harikumar K. B. "Potential therapeutic effects of curcumin, the anti-inflammatory agent, against neurodegenerative, cardiovascular, pulmonary, metabolic, autoimmune and neoplastic diseases." *International Journal of Biochemistry and Cell Biology* 2009; 41(1): 40–59

22 Chandran B. and Goel A. "A randomized, pilot study to assess the efficacy and safety of curcumin in patients with active rheumatoid arthritis." *Phytotherapy Research* November 2012; 26(11): 1719–25

23 Marini A., et al. "Pycnogenol effects on skin elasticity and hydration coincide with increased gene expressions of collagen type 1 and hyaluronic acid synthase in women." *Skin Pharmacology and Physiology* 2012; 25(2): 86–92

24 Tixier J. M., Godeau G., Robert A. M. and Hornebeck W. "Evidence by in vivo and in vitro studies that binding of pycnogenols to elastin

affects its rate of degradation by elastases." *Biochemical Pharmacology* December 15, 1984; 33 (24): 3933–9

Chapter 4

1   Stevenson S. and Thornton J. "Effect of estrogens on skin aging and the potential role of SERMs." *Clinical Interventions in Aging* September 2007; 2(3): 283–297

2   Dunn L. B., et al. "Does estrogen prevent skin aging? Results from the First National Health and Nutrition Examination Survey NHANES 1." *Archives of Dermatology* March 1997; 133(3): 339–42

3   Weeks D. and Jones J. *The Superyoung* 1999; London: Hodder Paperbacks

4   Calvo E., et al. "Pangenomic changes induced by DHEA in the skin of postmenopausal women." *Journal of Steroid Biochemistry and Molecular Biology* December 2008; 112(4–5): 186–193

5   Rudman D., et al. "Impaired growth hormone secretion in the adult population: relation to age and adiposity." *Journal of Clinical Investigation* May 1981; 67(5): 1361–69

6   Peckham S., Lowery D. and Spencer S. "Are fluoride levels in drinking water associated with hypothyroidism prevalence in England? A large observational study of GP practice data and fluoride levels in drinking water." *Journal of Epidemiology and Community Health* February 24, 2015; [online] jech.bmj.com

7   Thyroid Patient Advocacy

8   Diabetes UK

9   Donga E., et al. "A single night of partial sleep deprivation induces insulin resistance in multiple metabolic pathways in healthy subjects." *Journal of Clinical Endocrinology Metabolism* June 2010; 95(6): 2963–8

10   Bionsen, November 2009

11   O'Connell S. G., Kincl L. D. and Anderson K. A. "Silicone wristbands as personal passive samplers." *Environmental Science and Technology* March 18, 2014; 48(6): 3327–35

12   Environmental Working Group. "Toxic chemicals found in minority cord blood" December 2, 2009 [online] www.ewg.org

13   Barrett E. S., et al. "Environmental exposure to di-2-ethylhexyl phthalate is associated with low interest in sexual activity in premenopausal women." *Hormones and Behaviour* November 2014; 66(5): 787–92

14   Grindler N. M., et al. "Persistent organic pollutants and early menopause in US women." *PLoS One* January 28, 2015; 10(1): e0116057

15   Rajapakse N., Silva E. and Kortenkamp A. "Combining xenoestrogens at levels below individual no-observed-effect concentrations dramatically enhances steroid hormone action." *Environmental Health Perspectives* September 2002; 110(9): 917–21

16   Gonzales G. F., Gasco M. and Lozada-Requena I. "Role of maca (Lepidium meyenii) consumption on serum interleukin-6 levels and health status in populations living in the Peruvian Central Andes over 4000 m of altitude." *Plant Foods for Human Nutrition* December 2013; 68(4): 347–51

17   Meissner H. O., Reich-Bilinska H., Mscisz A. and Kedzia B. "Therapeutic effects of pre-gelatinized maca (Lepidium Peruvianum Chacon) used as a non-hormonal alternative to HRT in perimenopausal women—Clinical Pilot Study." *International Journal of Biomedical Science* June 2006; 2(2): 143–59

18   Talbott S. M., Talbott J. A. and Pugh M. "Effect of Magnolia officinalis and Phellodendron amurense (Relora®) on cortisol and psychological mood state in moderately stressed subjects." *Journal of the International Society of Sports Nutrition* August 7, 2013; 10(1): 37

19   Kanaley J. A. "Growth hormone, arginine and exercise." *Current Opinion in Clinical Nutrition and Metabolic Care* January 2008; 11(1): 50–4

Chapter 5

1   Rohrich R. J. and Pessa J. E. "The fat compartments of the face: anatomy and clinical implications for cosmetic surgery." *Plastic and Reconstructive Surgery* June 2007; 119(7): 2219–27

2   Grover R. "Prospective longitudinal study of aging in 118 women over 9 years using objective measurements reveals the concept of aging

Spurts" Presented at the International Master Course on aging Skin (IMCAS), January 2010, Paris

3   Shaw R. B. Jr., et al. "Aging of the mandible and its aesthetic implications" *Plastic and Reconstructive Surgery* January 2010; 125(1): 332–42

4   Peterson G., et al. "A novel fluorescent makeup methodology used to measure the cleansing efficacy of a sonic skin care brush." *Journal of the American Academy of Dermatology* February 2007; 56(2): supplement 2: AB38

5   Burke K. E. "Photodamage of the skin: protection and reversal with topical antioxidants." *Journal of Cosmetic Dermatology* July 2004; 3(3): 149–55

6   Blatt T., et al. "Modulation of oxidative stresses in human aging skin." *Gerontol Zeitschrift für Geriatrogie und* April 1999; 32(2): 83–8

7   Zhuang Y., Hou H., Zhao X., Zhang Z., Li B. "Effects of collagen and collagen hydrolysate from jellyfish (Rhopilema esculentum) on mice skin photoaging induced by UV irradiation." *Journal of Food Science*, August 2009; 74(6): H183–8

8   Bylka W., et al. "Centella asiatica in dermatology: an overview." *Phytotherapy Research* August 2014; 28(8): 1117–1124

9   Li Y. H., et al. "Protective effects of green tea extracts on photoaging and photoimmunosuppression." *Skin Research and Technology* August 2009; 15(3): 338–45

10 Gianeti M. D., Mercurio D. G. and Campos P. M. "The use of green tea extract in cosmetic formulations: not only an antioxidant active ingredient." *Dermatologic Therapy* May/June 2013; 26(3): 267–71

11 Seki M. "Treatment of adult acne with Pycnogenol." 2006; [online] www.pychogenol.com Horphag Research, Geneva

12 Randhawa M., et al. "One-year topical stabilized retinol treatment improves photodamaged skin in a double-blind, vehicle-controlled trial." *Journal of Drugs in Dermatology* March 1, 2015; 14(3): 271–80

13 Kang B. S., et al. "Antimicrobial activity of enterocins from Enterococcus faecalis SL-5 against Propionibacterium acnes, the causative agent in acne vulgaris and its therapeutic effect." *Journal of Microbiology* February 2009; 47(1): 101–9

14 Nair P. A. and Arora T. H. "Microneedling using Dermaroller a means of collagen induction therapy." *Gujarat Medical Journal* March 2014; (69)1: 24–7

15 Proksch E., et al. "Oral intake of specific bioactive collagen peptides reduces skin wrinkles and increases dermal matrix synthesis." *Skin Pharmacology and Physiology* 2014; 27(3): 113–9

16 Kawada C., et al. "Ingested hyaluronan moisturizes dry skin." *Nutrition Journal* July 2014; 13: 70

17 Kim H. H., et al. "Eicosapentaenoic acid inhibits UV-induced MMP-1 expression in human dermal fibroblasts." *Journal of Lipid Resarch* August 2005; 46(8): 1712–20

Chapter 6

1 Powell N. D., et al. "Social stress up-regulates inflammatory gene expression in the leukocyte transcriptome via beta-adrenergic induction of myelopoiesis." *Proceedings of the National Academy of Sciences of the USA.* October 8, 2013; 110(41): 16574–9

2 O'Donovan A., et al. "Stress appraisals and cellular aging. A key role of anticipatory threat in the relationship between psychological stress and telomere length." *Brain, Behaviour and Immunity* May 2012; 26(4): 573–9

3 Bhattacharya S. K., Bhattacharya A., Sairam K. and Ghosal S. "Anxiolytic-antidepressant activity of Withania somnifera glycowithanolides: an experimental study." *Phytomedicine* December 2000; 7(6): 463–9

4 Black D. S. et al. "Yogic meditation reverses NF-kB and IRF-related transcriptome dynamics in leukocytes of family dementia caregivers in a randomized controlled trial." *Psychoneuroendocrinology* March 2013; 38(3): 348–55

5 Handlin L., et al. "Short-term interaction between dogs and their owners: Effect on oxytocin, cortisol, insulin and heart rate—an exploratory study." *Anthrozoös* September 2011; 24(3): 301–15

6 Baron E., et al. "Effects of Sleep Quality on Skin Aging and Function." Presented at the International Investigative Dermatology Meeting, July 2013, Edinburgh

7   Sundelin T., et al. "Cues of fatigue: effects of sleep deprivation on facial appearance." *Sleep* September 1, 2013; 36(9): 1355–60

8   Irwin M. R., et al. "Sleep deprivation and activation of morning levels of cellular and genomic markers of inflammation." *Archives of International Medicine* September 18, 2006; 166(16): 1756–62

9   Wood B., et al. "Light level and duration of exposure determine the impact of self-luminous tablets on melatonin suppression." *Applied Ergonomics* March 2013: 44(2); 237–40

10   Liu A. G., et al. "Tart cherry juice increases sleep time in older adults with insomnia." *Journal of the Federation of American Societies for Experimental Biology* April 2014; 28(1): supplement 830.9

11   Cherkas L. F., et al. "The association between physical activity in leisure time and leukocyte telomere length." *Archives of International Medicine* January 28, 2008; 168(2): 154–8

12   Clake S. F., et al. "Exercise and associated dietary extremes impact on gut microbial diversity." *Gut* December 2014; 63(12): 1913–20

13   Tarnopolsky M. "Exercise as a countermeasure for aging: from mice to humans." Presented at the Annual Meeting of the American Medical Society for Sports Medicine, April 2014, New Orleans

14   Reynolds G. "Phys ed: how exercising keeps your cells young." *The New York Times* January 27, 2010; [online] well.blogs.nytimes.com

15   Keicolt-Glaser J. K., et al. "Yoga's impact on inflammation, mood and fatigue in breast cancer survivors: a randomized controlled trial." *Journal of Clinical Oncology* April 1, 2014; 32(10): 1040–9

16   Wen C. P., et al. "Minimum amount of physical activity of reduced mortality and extended life expectancy: a prospective cohort study." *The Lancet* October 1, 2011; 378(9798): 1244–53

17   Savela S., et al "Physical activity in midlife and telomere length measured in old age." *Experimental Gerontology* January 2013; 48(1): 81–84

18   Ludlow A. T., et al. "Relationship between physical activity level, telomere length and telomerase activity." *Medicine and Science in Sports and Exercise* October 2008; 40(10): 1764–71

19   Guyuron B., et al. "Factors contributing to the facial aging of identical twins." *Plastic and Reconstructive Surgery* April 2009; 123(4): 1321–31

20 Amros-Rudolph C. M., et al. "Malignant melanoma in marathon runners." *Archives of Dermatology* November 2006; 142(11): 1471–4
21 Langer E. J. *Counterclockwise* 2010; London: Hodder
22 Levy B. R., Slade M. D., Kunkel S. R. and Kasl S. V. "Longevity increased by positive self perceptions of aging." *Journal of Personality and Social Psychology* August 2002; 83(2): 261–70.
23 O'Donovan A. "Pessimism correlates with leucocyte telomere shortness and elevated interleukin-6 in post-menopausal women." *Brain, Behaviour and Immunity* May 2009; 23(4): 446–9
24 Levy B. and Leifheit-Limson E. "The stereotype-matching effect: greater influence on functioning when age stereotypes correspond to outcomes." *Psychology and Aging* March 2009; 24(1): 230–233
25 Becker C. B., Diedrichs P. C., Jankowski G. and Werchan C. "I'm not just fat, I'm old: has the study of body image overlooked old talk?" *Journal of Eating Disorders* February 21, 2013; 1: 6

Chapter 7

1 Whitehead R. D., Ozakinci G. and Perrett D. I. "Attractive skin coloration: harnessing sexual selection to improve diet and health." *Evolutionary Psychology* December 20, 2012; 10(5): 842–54
2 Nagata C., et al. "Association of dietary fat, vegetables and antioxidant macronutrients with skin aging in Japanese women." *British Journal of Nutrition* May 2010; 103(10): 1493–8
3 Di Noia J. "Defining powerhouse fruits and vegetables: a nutrient density approach." *Preventing Chronic Disease* June 5, 2014; 11: E95
4 BBC Television study. [online] www.bbc.co.uk/sn/humanbody/truthabout food/healthy/prebiotics.shtml
5 Bae J. Y., Kim J. L. and Kang Y. H. "Ellagic acid prevents ultraviolet radiation-induced chronic skin damage of skin cells in the hairless mice." Presented at the FASEB meeting, April 2009, New Orleans
6 Purba M. B., et al. "Skin Wrinkling: can food make a difference?" *Journal of the American College of Nutrition* February 2001; 20(1): 71–80
7 Daelos Z. D., Blair R. and Tabor A. "Oral soy supplementation and dermatology." *Cosmetic Dermatology* April 20, 2007; (4): 202–204

8   Palombo P., et al. "Beneficial long-term effects of combined oral/
    topical antioxidant treatment with the carotenoids lutein and
    zeaxanthin on human skin: a double-blind, placebo-controlled study."
    Skin Pharmacology and Physiology 2007; 20(4): 199–210

9   Kim S. R., et al. "Anti-wrinkle and anti-inflammatory effects of active
    garlic components and the inhibition of MMPs via NF-kB signalling."
    PLoS One September 16, 2013; 8(9): e738777

10 Chassaing B., et al. "Dietary emulsifiers impact the mouse gut
    microbiota promoting colitis and metabolic syndrome." *Nature* March
    5, 2015; 519(7541): 92–6

INDEX

A1 protein, in milk, 59
Aches, and inflammation, 97
Acid supplements, 43–44
Acne, 14; and milk, 67
Acne treatment face masks, 172–73
Acupuncture, 39
Adrenal fatigue, stages, 118–19
Adrenal function testing, 120
Adrenal glands, 117–18, 128
Advanced Glycation End Products
	(AGEs), 72
Age-reversing eating plan, 204–33;
	foods, recommended, 205–13;
	four-week plan, 213–23; meal
	creation, 223–29; recipes,
	234–61; shopping 229–30;
	summary, 230–33
Age-reversing lifestyle, 184–203,
	233; exercise, 196–200;
	positive thinking, 201–203;
	sleeping, 192–95; stress
	avoidance, 185–92
Aging. See Digest-aging
Aging signs, 8, 10
Alcohol: and hormone balancing,
	134; as ultimate ager, 39, 89;
	and Wine Face, 69–71
Algaes, 154, 211
Allergies, environmental, and
	inflammation, 92, 98
Allergies, food, 40, 49–50, 97–98
Alletess Laboratory IgG test, 55

Aloe vera juice, 46
Alpha-lipoic acid (oral
	supplement), 167–68
Amaranth, 207
Amylase (digestive enzyme),
	20–21, 44
Androgens, 115
Antibiotics: and dysbiosis, 24;
	limiting, 40
Antioxidant serums, 153–55
Antioxidants: and inflammation,
	105; in fruits and vegetables,
	recommended, 205–207, 223
Arnica, 39
Arsenic, 131
Artificial sweeteners, 73–74
Ascophyllum nodosum (fucowhite),
	154
Ashwagandha, and stress, 189
Avocado, 210

B vitamins: and hormone levels,
	17–18; and inflammation,
	103–104; production, 17; and
	stress, 187–88
Bacterial overgrowth, 30–31
Baker's yeast, 54
Baking soda test, 20
Basal cells, 147
Basic Nut Butter (recipe), 255–56
Beans, 209–10
Bedding, changing, 195

Berries, 207
Betaine HCl, 43–44
Bifidobacterium lactis (probiotic supplement), 42
Bile acid diarrhea (BAD), 36
Bile acids, and gut lining, 28
Bioidentical hormones, 136
Biotin, 17
Bisphenol-A (BPA), 130
Bittermelon, 138
Black cohosh, 137
Blastocystis hominis (parasite), 29
Blood glucose testing, 127–28
Blood tests, and food intolerance, 55–56
Bluish skin tone, 80
Body Mass Index (BMI), and inflammation, 100
Body position, while sleeping, 195
Body weight, and inflammation, 91–92, 99
Bone broth, 209; recipe, 239
Bones, in face, 149
Boswellia, 40, 107
Bottled water, 228
Breakfasts, 224; recipes, 234–37
Brewer's yeast, 54
Brows. *See* Eyebrows
BROWSK mnemonic, and gluten, 63
Buckwheat, 208
Buckwheat Bircher (recipe), 236
Butternut Squash Soup (recipe), 246–47

C-reactive protein (CRP), 91; testing, 94
Calcium d-glucarate, 135
Calcium sources, 67
Cancer, 37
Candida, 30
Castor oil packs, 64–65
"Catastrophizing," 189–90
Cauliflower Pizza (recipe), 252–53
CCP stages. *See* Clear stage; Correct stage; Protect stage
Celiac disease, 36, 62
Centella asiatica, 154
Chamomilla recutita (matricaria) extract, 152
Chasteberry extract, 137
Cheek area, on face, 78; make-up advice, 180
Chemical exposure, effect on hormones, 130–32, 134
Chemicals, in skincare products, 163
Chewing, and digestion, 18–19, 43
Chia Porridge (recipe), 234
Chia seeds, 211
Chickpeas with Spinach (recipe), 248–49
Childbirth, and dysbiosis, 23
Chili and Cauliflower Rice (recipe), 254–55
Chili Power Spicy Sauce (recipe), 256–57
Chilies, 212
Chin area, on face, 79
Cholestyramine, and bile acid diarrhea, 36

Cinnamon, 212
Cinnamon and Honey Face Mask
    (recipe), 173
Clarisonic brushes, 152
Cleanliness, and dysbiosis, 23–24
Cleansing and cleansers, 150–52;
    recommended, 169–70
Clear stage: Gut-Balancing CCP
    Plan, 38–42, 263; Hormone-
    Balancing CCP Plan, 133–35,
    265; Inflammation-Fighting
    CCP Plan, 96–100, 264;
    Skincare CCP Plan, 150–52
Coconut Milk (recipe), 260–61
Coconut oil, 211
Cod Provençale (recipe), 251
Co-enzyme Q10, 153–54
Coffee, 228
Collagen, 147, 148; and DHEA,
    117; marine, 154; oral
    supplement, 167
Color: of complexion, 79–81; of
    foods in diet, 140–41
Concealer, make-up advice, 178
Correct stage: Gut-Balancing CCP
    Plan, 42–44, 264; Hormone-
    Balancing CCP Plan, 135–38,
    266; Inflammation-Fighting
    CCP Plan, 101–105, 265;
    Skincare CCP Plan, 153–60
Cortisol, 52, 128–29; symptoms of
    high level, 129
Cow's milk. See Dairy products
COX-2 enzymes, 106, 107
Cravings, and food intolerances, 57
Creamy skin cleansers, 163

Curcumin, 105
Curried Brussels Sprouts Salad
    (recipe), 241–42
Cystitis, 76
Cytokines, 83, 84–85, 90, 91, 106
Dairy Face, 65–68; symptoms,
    65–66
Dairy Face Mask (recipe), 174
Dairy products: and food
    intolerance, 53, 59, 88; and
    hormone balancing, 133; as
    ultimate ager, 39, 88
Dark skin tone, 80
Defecation, ideal, 34
Deglycyrrhizinated licorice (DGL),
    46
Delayed allergy syndrome, 51
Delta-6 desaturase, 89, 106
Dermatitis herpetiformis, 65
Dermis, 147
Desquamation, 147
Devil's claw, 40
DHEA (dehydroepiandrosterone),
    117–21
Diarrhea, severe, as symptom, 36
Dietary fats. See Fats, dietary
Dietary oils. See Oils, dietary
Digest-aging, 4–5, 9–12, 15–35;
    checklists, 9–11
Digestion, poor, 18–22
Digestive enzymes, 44
Digestive system, size, 13
Diindolylmethane (DIM), 64,
    137–38
Dinners, recipes, 242–55

Dioxins, 130–31
Dips and mixes, recipes, 255–58
"Dirty hormones," 25, 114, 125;
    fixers, 206
DNA, 86; and UV rays, 161, 193
Drinks, recipes, 259–61
Dysbiosis, 22–26; and gut lining,
    28

"Eat the rainbow" concept, 140–41
Eating out, 226
Echium oil, 103
Eggs, 209; and food intolerance,
    54
"80:20 life" concept, 230–31
Elastin, 147, 148
Elimination, 33–34
Elimination diet, 54–55
Endocrine disruptors, 114, 130–32
Environmental allergies, and
    inflammation, 92, 98
Enzyme boosters, and
    inflammation, 106–107
Enzyme levels, 20–22
Epidermis, 146–47
Equipment, kitchen, 229
Estrogen, 113–17; dominance,
    115; imbalance symptoms,
    116
Exercise, 196–200; and hGh, 123;
    and hormone balancing, 135;
    mistakes, 198–200; types,
    197–98
Extrinsic aging, 143

Eye area, on face: between eyes,
    76–77; make-up advice,
    180–82; under eyes, 77–78
Eye creams, 158
Eye make-up remover, 150–51;
    recommended, 169
Eyebrow area, on face, 77; make-
    up advice, 180
Eyeshadow, make-up advice, 181

Face care products: homemade,
    170–75; recommended,
    169–70
Face-freezing, 145–46
Face-mapping, and body
    symptoms, 74–81
Facial bones, 149
Facial contouring, make-up advice,
    178–79
Facial massage, 159–60
Facial oils, 162–63
Facial wipes, 163
Fats, dietary: healthy, 101–103;
    and inflammation, 89–91;
    recommended, 210–11;
    reducing, 96–97
Fats, facial, 149
Fenugreek, 138
Ferulic acid, 154
Fiber, 42–43; insoluble, 34, 43;
    soluble, 43
Filler injections, 145–46
Fish oil supplements, 102–103,
    168
5-LOX enzymes, 106, 107
Flaxseeds and flaxseed oil, 211

Folic acid, and stress, 188
Follicle-stimulating hormone (FSH), 116
Food additives (E466 and E433), 231
Food allergies, 40, 49–50, 97–98
Food diaries, 56–57
Food intolerance, 40, 49–60; symptoms, 58; tests, 54–57
Food plan, 213–23
Food-processing methods, 59
Food shopping, 229–30
Forehead area, on face, 76
Foundation, make-up advice, 176–78
"Four Faces" of aging, 48, 60–74; Dairy Face, 65–68; Gluten Face, 61–65; Sugar Face, 71–74; Wine Face, 69–71
Free radicals, 51
Fructose, 73, 74; malabsorption, 74
Fucowhite (*Ascophyllum nodosum*), 154
Fungus, 30

Gamma-linoleic acid (GLA), 106–107
Garlic, 212
Glucose Tolerance Test, 127–28
Glutamine, 46
Gluten: and celiac disease, 36; and food intolerance, 53, 59, 62, 88; giving up, 63–64; and gut lining, 28–29; and hormone balancing, 133; as ultimate ager, 39, 88
Gluten Face, 61–65; symptoms, 61
Glycation, 72, 126
Glycemic index, 89
Glycolic acid, 151, 152
Glycyrrhizin, 46
Gotu Kola, 154
Grains, recommended, 207–208, 223
"Green detoxifiers," 139
Green Juices (recipe), 259–60
Green tea, 154–55
Greenish skin tone, 80
Gut: bacteria, 13–14, 17–26; and emotions, 14–15; and stress, 15
Gut-Balancing CCP Plan, 37–47, 49, 88–89, 96; clearing stage, 38–42; correction stage, 42–44; protection stage, 45–47
Gut-inflammation, 48–49

Hara Hachi Bu (meal satisfaction), 227
Harissa Mix (recipe), 258
Healthy Curry (recipe), 245–46
Helicobacter pylori, 46
Helix aspersa Müller, 156
Herbs, recommended, 212–13, 223
hGh (human growth hormone), 121–23
High-intensity interval training (HIIT), 197

Hormone-Balancing CCP Plan, 132–41; clear stage, 133–35; correct stage, 135–38; protect stage, 138–41

Hormone profile test, 136

Hormones: and hormonal imbalance, 33, 109–41; and adrenal glands, 117–21; aging, 126–32; balancing plan, 132–41; and chemical exposure, 130–32, 134; and pigmentation, 110–12; and stress, 186; youth boosters, 113–26. *See also* "Dirty hormones"

Hyaluronic acid, 52, 147, 148, 155; oral supplement, 168

Hydration, 227–28; of skin, 155–56

Hydrogenated fats, 91

Hydrolyzed collagen, 167

"Hygiene hypothesis," 60

Hyperbaric oxygen infusion, 166

Hypochlorhydria, 20–22

Hypodermis, 149

IgE (antibody) reactions, 51

IGF-1 (hormone), 121

IgG (antibody): reactions, 51–54; testing, 55

Inflamm-aging. *See* Inflammation, chronic

Inflammation, chronic, 22, 82–108; causes, 87–95; and stress, 186; testing, 94; word origin, 85

Inflammation-Fighting CCP Plan, 95–108; clear stage, 96–100; correct stage, 101–105; protect stage, 105–108

Inflammatory bowel disease, 37

Insulin, 88, 121, 126; and insulin resistance, 126–28; and pigmentation, 111

Insulin resistance, 126–28; symptoms, 127; testing, 127–28

Interleukin-1 alpha (IL-1α), 85

Intestines, and digestion, 20–22

Iodine, 125–26

Irritable bowel syndrome (IBS), 31

Isoflavones, 117, 140

"Itis" conditions, 94, 98

Juices, recipes, 259–60

Kale and Apple Salad (recipe), 240–41

Kimchi, 212–13

Kirtan Kriya meditation, 190–91

Kitchen gadgets, 229

L'Arginine, 138

Lactobacillus family, 25, 42

Lactose intolerance, 56, 66

Langer, Ellen, 201

Large intestine, and digestion, 22

Leaky gut, 16, 26–31

LED skin treatments, 165–66

Legumes, 209–10

Leukotrienes, 83–84, 90

Light audit, of sleeping area, 194

Lima Bean Hummus (recipe), 244
Linoleic acid, 90
Lipase (digestive enzyme), 20–21, 44
Lip area, on face, 78–79; make-up advice, 182–83
Liquor, and Wine Face, 69–71. *See also* Alcohol
"Listen to your body" concept, 231
Liver, 32; attention to, 139
"Low T3 Syndrome," 125
Lunches, 224–25; recipes, 238–42

Maca, 136–37
Make-up: advice, 175–83; and exercise, 200; recommended, 169–70
Malabsorption/maldigestion, 16–19; defined, 18
Marine collagen, 154
Massage, of face, 159–60
Mastic gum, 46
Mechnikov, Ilya, 15
Medical skin needling, 164–65
Meditation, 190–92
Melanin, 111, 147
Melasma (pigmentation), 111–12
Melatonin, 129, 193–94; supplements, 194
Menthol-based pain relief products, 40
Mercury, 131
Meridians, 75
Methylisothiazolinone (MI), in facial wipes, 163
Mexican Peppers (recipe), 247–48

Microbiome/microbiota, and dysbiosis, 23, 25
Microdermabrasion/peels, 166–67
Micronutrients, absorption, 19
Milk, cow's, and food intolerances, 53, 59. *See also* Dairy products
Milk thistle, 139
Milk, non-dairy, 68; recipes, 260–61
Mindfulness, 190; in eating, 232–33
Minerals, absorption, 17
Minted Quinoa (recipe), 239–40
Moisturizing and moisturizers, 155–56; recommended, 169
Monounsaturated fats, 89, 101
Mucosa-boosting foods, 45
Mustard Dressing (recipe), 258

Natural supplements, and hormone balancing, 136–38
NF-kappa-B, 95
Niacin, and stress, 188
Non-celiac gluten sensitivity, 62
Nose area, on face, 78; make-up advice, 179
Nut Milks (recipe), 260
Nuts and nut butters, 211; recipe, 255–56

Oils, dietary, recommended, 210, 211, 223
Oily fish, 209
"Old speak" concept, 203
Olives and olive oil, 211

Omega-3 fats, 89, 90, 96–97, 101–103, 106
Omega-6 fats, 89, 90, 96–97, 106
ORAC values, 228
Oral antioxidants (supplements), 168
Organic foods, 41–42
Organic wines, 71

Pain medications, 39
Pains, and inflammation, 97
Paleness, 80
Pancreatic insufficiency, 21–22
Pantothenic acid, and stress, 188
Papaya and Avocado Scrub (recipe), 173–74
Parasites, 29, 41
Partially hydrogenated fats, 91
Perfect Skin Dip (recipe), 256
Permeability tests, and leaky gut, 28
Petroleum-based skincare products, 163
Pets, as stress relievers, 192
Phosphatidylserine, and stress, 189
Phthalates, 131
Pigmentation, 110–12
Plant stem cells, 154, 158
Polyunsaturated fats, 90
Positive thinking, 201–203
Poultry, 209
Power Porridges (recipe), 234–35
Prebiotic Power Bowl (recipe), 243
Prebiotics, 45, 207
Prediabetes, 127

Probiotics, 15–16; and dysbiosis, 26; supplements, 42; topical, 157
Processed foods, avoiding, 231
Professional skincare treatments, 164–67
Progesterone, 115, 129
Pro-resolution molecules, 101
Prostaglandins, 83, 84–85, 90
Protease (digestive enzyme), 20–21, 44
Protect stage: Gut-Balancing CCP Plan, 45–47, 264; Hormone-Balancing CCP Plan, 138–41, 266; Inflammation-Fighting CCP Plan, 105–108, 265; Skincare CCP Plan, 161–68
Protein absorption, 17, 19
Proteins, recommended, 208–10, 223
Pupillary light reflex test, for adrenal function, 120
Pycnogenol, 107, 155

Quinoa, 208

Radio frequency treatment, 166
Recipes, homemade skincare products, 170–75
Recipes, meals, 234–61; breakfast, 234–37; dinner, 242–55; dips and mixes, 255–58; drinks, 259–61; lunch, 238–42
Red meat, 210
Red wine, 70–71
Reddish skin tone, 79–80

Relora, 137
Retin-A (tretinoin), 156–57
Retinols, 156–57
Rhodiola, and stress, 188–89
Rice, 208
Rosacea, 31

Salicylic acid, 151–52
Salt, 213
Saturated fats, 89–90
Seasonal eating, 232
Seasonings, recommended,
    212–13, 223
Sedentary lifestyle, and
    inflammation, 94–95
Seeds, recommended, 211, 223
SeHCAT scan, 36
Selenium, 125
Serotonin, 14
Serving size, 225
Sexy Skin Salad (recipe), 240
Short-chain fatty acids (SCFAs), 22
Skin, 143–44; ages, 144–46;
    cleansing, 150–52; layers, 143,
    146–49; tone, 79–81
Skin-Boosting Salad Dressing
    (recipe), 257
Skincare CCP Plan, 150–62; clean
    stage, 150–52; correct stage,
    153–60; protect stage, 161–62
Skincare products: to avoid, 162–
    64; recommended, 169–70
Skincare treatments, professional,
    164–67

Sleeping, 192–95; and hormone
    balancing, 135; and
    inflammation, 93, 99
Slippery elm, 46–47
Small intestinal bacterial
    overgrowth (SIBO), 30–31
Small intestine, and digestion,
    20–22
Smoking, and inflammation,
    93–94
Smooth Skin Smoothie (recipe),
    236–37
Snacks, 226–27
Snail mucus, as moisturizer, 155
    –56
Soy products, 210; and food
    intolerance, 53
Spiced Lentils (recipe), 244–45
Spiced Noodle Soup (recipe), 250
Spices: and inflammation, 104–
    105; recommended, 212–13,
    223
Spicy Soup (recipe), 238
Stages. See Clear stage; Correct
    stage; Protect stage
Starling, Ernest, 113
Stir-Fry Skin Magic (recipe), 243
Stomach, and digestion, 19–20
Stomach acid levels: balancing,
    43–44; low, 20
Stools: ideal, 34; tests, 41
Stratum corneum, 146–47
Stress, 40; and aging connection,
    185–92; and hormone
    balancing, 135; and
    inflammation, 93; managing,

187–92; and pigmentation, 111
Stuffed Peppers (recipe), 249
Sugar: cravings, 73–74; and hormone balancing, 133–34; as ultimate ager, 39, 72, 88–89
Sugar Face, 71–74; symptoms, 71
Sulfites, in wine, 71
Sunglasses, 161–62
Sunscreens, 161, 162, 200; recommended, 170
Super Skin Mix (recipe), 257
Superfood power ups, 235
Supplements, 38. *See also specific supplements*
Sweating, 139–40
Sweet Potato Cakes (recipe), 235–36

T3 (triiodothyronine), 125
T4 (thyroxine), 125
Tea, 228
Teff, 208
Telomeres, 86–87, 89
Temperature test, for thyroid function, 124–25
Testosterone, 115, 129
Tests: for adrenal function, 120; for bile acid diarrhea, 36; for candida, 30; for food intolerance, 55–56; for glucose levels, 127–28; hormone profile, 136; for IgG antibodies, 55–56; for inflammation, 94; for insulin resistance, 127–28; for leaky gut, 28; for stomach acid, 20; for thyroid function, 124–25; at-home, 20, 120, 124
Thiamine, and stress, 188
Thornfeldt, Carl, 85
Thyroid hormones, 123–26
Thyroid stimulating hormone (TSH), 125
Tiger Balm, 40
Tight junctions, and leaky gut, 27
Tilbury, Charlotte: make-up advice, 175–83
Toxins, in liver, 32
Traditional Chinese Medicine (TCM), and faces, 60, 74–81
Trans fats, 91
Tumor-necrosis factor alpha (TNF-α), 84–85, 107
Turmeric, 170, 213
Turmeric and Chamomile Face Mask (recipe), 172–73
Turmeric Eggs (recipe), 237
Turmeric mask (recipe), 170–72
12-week plan, 263–66
Tyrosinase, 111, 112

"Ultimate agers," 39, 96; and inflammation, 88–89; and hormone balancing, 133–34. *See also* Alcohol; Dairy products; Gluten; Sugar
UV rays, 85, 161
UVB rays, 161

Variety in diet, importance, 231

Vegetables, recommended, 205–206
Vegetarians: and digestive enzymes, 44; and omega-3 fats, 103
Veggie Bowl (recipe), 242
Vitamin A, 68, 168; and inflammation, 103
Vitamin B. *See* B vitamins
Vitamin C, 153, 168; and inflammation, 104
Vitamin D, and inflammation, 104
Vitamin E, 168
Vitamins: absorption, 17, 21; and inflammation, 103–104. *See also specific vitamins*

Waist measurements, and inflammation, 99–100
Walking, 198
Water, 227; bottled, 228
Weight, and inflammation, 91–92, 99
Whole-body vibration, 198
Wine, 70–71
"Wine and dine" area, on face, 77
Wine Face, 69–71; symptoms, 69

Xenoestrogens, 114

Yeast, and food intolerance, 54
Yellowish skin tone, 80
Yoga, 197–98

DR. NIGMA'S MAGIC NUTRITIONAL SUPPLEMENTS

My mission is to offer results-driven nutritional supplements that enhance your health, wellness and beauty, giving you radiant and younger-looking skin from within.

As not all vitamins, probiotics, minerals and amino acids are created equal, I created my own line of ingestible beauty. The right combination of nutritional supplements should be an essential part of your skincare routine and the bonus is that these nutrients work synergistically from within to give you outer glow, reduce overall inflammation and help you reach optimal wellness. You can find these through many online retailers, including:

- Healthydoc.com
- www.thebeautyagenda.uk
- youngLDN.com
- Nordstrom.com
- Net-a-Porter.com
- Goop.com
- Violetgrey.com
- Thirteenlune.com
- victoriahealth.com
- oxygenboutique.com
- Shanidarden.com
- Figface.com
- Tacha.es
- Georgialouise.com
- lacandco.com
- Amazon.com

Vitamin C Cocktail: A powder that packs a powerful combination of PureWay-C™ patented liposomal technology for optimal bioavailability, zinc, VitaBerry® Superfruit Blend—a powerful formulation of high-ORAC super fruit, and phosphatidylcholine (PC)—naturally occurring in the human body; PC is an essential phospholipid and component of cell membranes. Up to 90 percent of the vitamin C (ascorbic acid) in this product is absorbed into the cells without being excreted as with other generic vitamin C products.

B Famous: An extremely potent formula delivering a combination of all the B vitamins that are present in their active form, allowing the body to have the highest available absorption.

Beauty in a Bottle: This supplement is incredible for optimal hair, skin and nail health. As a bonus, it's great for the immune system and hormone health. Vitamins, minerals, amino acids and other nutrients, such as ingestible hyaluronic acid, work in synergy, helping to rebuild collagen and keratin formation. I use this as a multivitamin for overall beauty and wellness.

Beauty Collagen Cocktail: This powder is packed with a powerful combination of cutting-edge bioavailable marine collagen, branched-chain amino acids, antioxidants, electrolytes and probiotics to give you everything your skin needs to glow from within.

Healthy Flora Probiotics: Each capsule is packed with a researched blend of probiotics (including *Lactobacillus acidophilus* DDS1 strain, a mix of bifidobacteria and grape seed extract) to improve digestion, overall gut health and skin health.

Vitamin D Sun: A powerful supplement packed with high-potency D3 with K1 and K2 that work together to maximize the absorption of vitamin D. Vitamin D helps reduce overall inflammation with the bonus of promoting healthy skin cells.

ACKNOWLEDGMENTS

My sincerest thank you to all my patients throughout the world for their commitment toward their health and wellness; you inspire me.

Thank you Amelia and Jamie Dornan for testing my recipes, and to Jeremy Piven for inspiring and reminding me to exercise and meditate to find my center.

To the gracious and gorgeous Sienna Miller, thank you for spreading the word about my work to your loved ones.

To the beautiful Kate Bosworth for being such a supportive friend and cheerleader; your advice and support has helped me immensely—thank you!

To the shining star, Stella McCartney, for all your lovely gifts to me and my team at Healthydoc and all your referrals and your ongoing support.

To the glorious Rosie Huntington-Whiteley and Jason Statham, thank you for spreading the news on my book worldwide. I'm so thrilled you love the book! You both rock!

Thank you to the beautiful-inside-and-out couple Penelope Cruz and Javier Bardem for spreading the word about my work and my book; it means so much to me that it has changed your life. Many thanks also to Charlotte Tilbury for her amazing makeup tricks and tips.

My friends whom have been my rock throughout this journey. I would like to thank my loving friends, Judy Joo, Imran Amed, Dr. Michelle Sayour and Dr. Keith Berkowitz, for supporting me and building the awareness about my field of medicine as a naturopathic doctor and as an anti-aging skin expert. A special thank you to my lifelong friends in Vancouver for your unconditional love: you know who you are.

I'm so grateful to my beautiful family: my mom, Parin; my dad, Mohamed; my sister, Waheeda; and my adorable dogs, Dante and the late Mimi —for your commitment, guidance and unconditional love.

To the honorable Helen for her perseverance and reassurance.

Thank you to the fabulous team at Penguin Random House for approaching me to write a book—it has been an incredible journey from that day forward—and to Ulysses Press, which published the book in the United States.

To all the naturopathic doctors and colleagues worldwide, I salute you for working in a field of medicine that is the crucial piece of completing the full spectrum of optimal health and wellness.

To my favorite doctors and healthcare practitioners who have been like teachers to me: naturopathic doctors Dr. Kelly Farnsworth and Dr. Gaetano Morello for being instrumental in my being the doctor I am today and for their commitment to naturopathic and integrative medicine and patient care.

ABOUT THE AUTHOR

Dr. Nigma Talib is a world-renowned naturopathic doctor, aesthetician and leading authority on holistic health. She has opened clinics in the UK, US and Canada, and currently practices in Los Angeles, California.

Her unique approach combines natural and complementary therapies such as acupuncture, Traditional Chinese Medicine and homeopathy with innovative laboratory testing, nutritional biochemistry, internal support and pioneering face treatments. With this holistic and bespoke approach to each client, she works to identify, address and heal underlying causes of disease rather than simply suppressing symptoms. Her areas of expertise range from premature aging and chronic skin problems to digestive complaints, infertility, hormonal disorders and sleep disorders.